GU00983118

SEXUALITY, NURSING
AND
HEALTH

Christine Webb
BA MSc PhD SRN RSCN RNT

Principal Lecturer in Nursing
Bristol Polytechnic

An H M + M Nursing Publication

JOHN WILEY & SONS
Chichester · New York · Brisbane · Toronto · Singapore

© John Wiley & Sons Ltd 1985

H M + M Publishers is an imprint of John Wiley & Sons Ltd

Library of Congress Cataloging-in-Publication Data:

Webb, Christine.
  Sexuality, nursing, and health.

  (An H M + M nursing publication)
  Bibliography: p.
  Includes index.
  1. Nurse and patient. 2. Sick—Sexual behavior.
3. Nurse and physician. 4. Sexism in medicine. 5. Sex.
I. Title. II. Series: HM+M nursing publication.
[DNLM: 1. Nurse–Patient Relations. 2. Nursing
Process. 3. Sex Behavior—nurses' instruction.
BF 692 W365s]
RT87.S49W43 1985   610.73   85–13627
ISBN 0 471 90818 5

British Library Cataloguing in Publication Data:

Webb, Christine
  Sexuality, nursing and health.
  1. Nurse and patient 2. Sick—Sexual behavior
  I. Title
  610.73'06'99   RT86.3

  ISBN 0 471 90818 5

Printed and bound in Great Britain

SEXUALITY,
NURSING
AND
HEALTH

Contents

Preface

This book grows out of my experience as a nurse who has studied sociology and carried out three research projects in the field of gynaecological nursing. Working as a nurse and spending many hours interviewing hysterectomy patients and gynaecology nurses led me to realise how much sexuality has been ignored in nursing and in health care in general. The women patients I interviewed told me of their fears and misapprehensions as they faced gynaecological surgery, and how little information they had been given to help them understand their experience and take an active role in controlling their own health. Gynaecology nurses spoke in my research interviews with them of the special emotional needs of their patients, revealing as they did so both a great wish to help and a lack of sound knowledge on which to draw.

Being a woman in nursing at a time when traditional ideas of what it is to be a woman or a man are being increasingly challenged has helped me to become aware that sexuality is an important factor in relationships between nurses, doctors and patients, and in the development of the nursing profession itself. The subordinate status of nurses in relation to doctors is a product of a long history of health care going back beyond Florence Nightingale. But her struggle to establish nursing as a profession for women and the later battles over state registration consolidated the division of labour between the sexes which had developed in wider society. Just as these divisions have undesirable consequences in human relations in general, so do they in health care, and the quality of care that patients receive is adversely affected as a result. Health workers cannot make the fullest contribution of which they are capable because of stereotyped judgements about who should do which kinds of work and how individuals should relate to one another. Patients and clients are also disadvantaged by stereotyping and their standards of health and styles of living are affected by ideas about sexuality.

Because of my experiences, I wanted to write a book for nurses which would discuss issues of sexuality in relation both to patients and clients who receive care and to those who give care, whether they are professionals or lay carers. I wanted to use a research-based approach and to present research findings about sexuality in a critical way, evaluating conflicting points of view and the research methods used to produce the 'evidence'. As well as being 'research-minded', I wanted the book to use a nursing process approach and give concrete examples of how theoretical ideas about sexuality were highly relevant in day-to-day nursing care.

This book is the result of my efforts, and I hope it will be useful to nurses studying at basic and post-basic levels. Whilst my own work has been principally in women's health, the book looks at how issues of sexuality are relevant to all patients and clients and so it should be meaningful to those in a wide range of specialities. It is intended to provide general information which all nurses can use in their work, and to serve as a foundation for those going on to specialise in fields where sexual counselling is carried out, such as some kinds of gynaecological, family planning and psychiatric nursing.

Section One explores theories of sexuality, looking at biological, psychological and sociological explanations of sexual differences, social roles, health and illness. We shall see that there are more similarities between women and men than there are differences, and that ideas of appropriate female and male behaviour have become stereotypes which can be harmful to the health of all of us. Whatever the origins of today's social arrangements for family life and work, new ideas offer possibilities for more fulfilling and healthier ways of living for women, men and children.

Section Two goes on to link these ideas to patients' and clients' needs in relation to sexuality and to examine how a whole range of illnesses, disabilities and treatments can affect these needs. Not only patients and clients, but also those who care for them, will feel the influence of these caring roles on their sexuality. We shall see how community care policies are based on assumptions about sexuality, and how these policies affect informal carers, who are mainly women.

Section Three will take up these themes in relation to nurses and nursing. We shall see how sexuality has come to be ignored and how the role of nurses in assessing, planning, giving and evaluating care to take account of sexuality might be developed. Finally, it will be suggested that the question of sexuality will continue to be a fundamental one for nurses as social changes in the areas of gender, sexual divisions of labour, and rising expectations for standards of care demand new approaches to nursing which place sexuality firmly on the agenda.

CHRISTINE WEBB
January 1985

Acknowledgements

So many people have helped me directly and indirectly to develop my ideas about the topics discussed in this book that I cannot name them all, but the patients and nurses who took part in my research projects deserve a special word of thanks. My gratitude also goes to colleagues at the Bristol & Weston School of Nursing and to Alex Massey, Jan Smith and Jackie Wall, who read and made valuable comments on the first draft. Angela King skilfully drew Figure 2.1 and the cartoons in Chapters 2 & 3, and Viv Quillan kindly gave permission to use her cartoon which appears in Chapter 4. Figure 3.1 is reproduced by permission of Virago Press Ltd.

CW

Theories
of
Sexuality

CHAPTER 1

What is Sexuality?

What is sexuality, and how is it relevant to nursing care? Answering the first question is not easy, as many writers imply when they talk about the topics included under the term 'sexuality' but avoid giving an actual definition. But a definition is important because it enables us to answer the second question about the relevance of sexuality to nursing, both to nurses themselves and to the care they give.

Rosemary Hogan (1980) in her book *Human Sexuality: A Nursing Perspective* considers that sexuality is "much more than the sex act.... the quality of being human, all that we are as men and women.... encompassing the most intimate feelings and deepest longings of the heart to find meaningful relationships". Straight-away we can see that sexuality is much more the biological side of sex acts, and is also more all-encompassing than the emotional aspects of sexual relationships. It involves the totality of being human, as another nursing writer, Lion (1982), shows in her book *Human Sexuality in Nursing Process*. For her, sexuality includes "all those aspects of the human being that relate to being boy or girl, woman or man, and is an entity subject to lifelong dynamic change. Sexuality reflects our human character not solely our genital nature".

'Self-concept' is a useful notion when thinking about sexuality because it enables us to understand the interaction of biological, psychological and social influences on how we see ourselves. People with positive self-concepts respect themselves and consider themselves worthwhile beings, not necessarily better than

3

others, but at least equal to them. In other words, they have high self-esteem. Conversely, low self-esteem and a negative self-concept come from self-dissatisfaction, self-rejection and even self-contempt (Stone, Cohen & Adler 1979).

Our basic self-concept develops as part of our personality and results from how we think other people view us. If others like us and show this by being friendly, interested and wanting to spend time with us, this builds up our positive self-concept and self-esteem. But if people avoid us, criticise us and are unfriendly, this also tells us something about ourselves and tends to lower our self-esteem. Basic self-concept is therefore modified by the responses of significant others and by particular events. Self-esteem is built up or confirmed by successfully coping with a stressful event such as taking an examination, moving house, being ill or having a bereavement. On the other hand, it may be damaged if the outcome of a traumatic event is interpreted negatively. The self-concept, then, is a social phenomenon, and supportive networks of family and friends play a vital role in validating self-worth when challenges threaten our self-esteem (Norbeck 1981).

'Gender' is the term used to describe these social aspects of sexuality, and the word 'sex' is usually reserved for the biological aspects, although we shall see how difficult it is to separate these aspects in real life (Oakley 1972).

Enough has been said already about sexuality to allow us to begin to answer the second question asked earlier, which was 'How is sexuality relevant to nursing care?' Ideas about holistic nursing which underpin the nursing process are clearly incomplete unless they include such a basic part of humanity as sexuality in care planning. The aim of taking sexuality into account in health care, according to the World Health Organisation (Mace, Bannerman & Burton 1974) is to promote sexual health. This is defined as:

1 A capacity to enjoy and control sexual and reproductive behaviour in accordance with a social and personal ethic.
2 Freedom from fear, shame, guilt, false beliefs, and other psychological factors inhibiting sexual response and impairing sexual relationships.
3 Freedom from organic disorders, diseases, and deficiencies that interfere with sexual and reproductive functions.

This definition includes aspects of sexuality relating to sexual activity in health, disability or illness. People who are ill will suffer to some degree from general feelings of malaise and tiredness.

They will not be able to distinguish between the physical tiredness of slow movements, heavy limbs and so on, and the accompanying emotional weariness and lack of enthusiasm which may be on a continuum from slight impairment and loss of zest, right through to pathological depression. At the same time, they are less able to carry out their usual social roles and fulfill their responsibilities at work and at home, which may move them further towards the depressed end of the continuum, and add more physical symptoms such as change in bowel or sleeping habits. If people are unable to meet social expectations through illness or disability, they may feel guilt, shame or embarrassment, and other people's reactions may reinforce these feelings. The self-concept, including sexuality, will clearly be disturbed too, with possible detrimental effects on self-esteem. Biopsychosocial influences on sexuality are thus so closely intertwined that it is impossible to unravel them.

The nature of an illness or disability will affect the person's response. A short, minor illness may induce a loss of self-esteem which will soon be regained. But a long, major or permanently disabling condition may change the self-concept irrevocably, making the person feel socially and sexually unattractive, inadequate and depressed.

Stage in the life-cycle is another factor which will affect the sexual implications of disability or illness for the sexual self-concept. Manifestations of sexuality vary through the stages of human development. For example, in our culture children learn about expectations of sex-role behaviour by as early as two years of age and have preferences for dressing and playing based on what they have learned (Oakley 1972). By the teenage years these differences are very well developed and genital sexual behaviour assumes great importance. In adulthood, forming more permanent sexual relationships, having children, and working life involve sexuality, and as people grow older the physical changes of ageing begin. Sexuality is revealed and experienced differently during these various phases of the life cycle, and thus the interplay of illness or disability and sexuality will also be different.

The setting in which care is given is another problematic variable, whether we consider an institution or clients' homes. Clients may not have separate rooms, or may sleep in a room which is shared with others during the day or night-time. They may be dependent on carers for maintaining their personal appearance, choosing and buying clothes, and arranging their hair, as well as a range of other activities in which we are usually autonomous. Their social contacts may be extremely limited, and here again lack of privacy may inhibit being relaxed and spontaneous with others. In both institutional and non-institutional settings, possibilities of expressing sexuality in all its dimensions may therefore be seriously curtailed.

Stuart & Sundeen's interpretation is concise but comprehensive in putting these ideas together to form a definition of sexuality and to see how fundamental this is to the totality of person in all aspects of life. They state that:

> "Sexuality is an integral part of the whole person. Human beings are sexual in every way, all the time. To a large extent human sexuality determines who we are. It is an integral factor in the uniqueness of every person."
> (Stuart & Sundeen 1979)

Once this broad definition is accepted, enormous numbers of new questions are opened up about sexuality in health, illness, disability and nursing. In the next three chapters, sexuality will be explored from the different perspectives of biology, psychology and sociology in order to develop further the many implications of sexuality for health care and for nursing.

CHAPTER 2

Biology and Sexuality

Most people would agree that there are biological differences between the sexes, but the size and importance of these differences would be a matter of greater debate. We shall start the discussion by examining sex differences and sexual development over the life cycle, going on to consider various biological explanations for these. Our aim will be to evaluate these explanations and come to a judgement of the relative importance of biological differences in our lives as sexual beings.

SEXUAL DIFFERENTIATION BEFORE BIRTH

During the first seven weeks of intra-uterine life the internal and external genital organs of all fetuses are identical. Embryos which will develop as females have two X chromosomes and genetic males have one X and one Y chromosome. The Y chromosome has virtually no functional genes, whereas the X chromosome has many, including those producing colour-blindness, haemophilia, and some forms of heart defect and mental handicap. Most of these are recessive, so that if they are paired with another gene of a different type they will cause no damage, and in females, having two X chromosomes usually leads to the second one cancelling out the harmful effects. In males the Y chromosome does not have this effect, and this leads to the formation of sex-linked characteristics such as colour-blindness (Archer & Lloyd 1982). This increased possibility of congenital defects in males helps to account for the fact that, although more males than females are conceived, the number of surviving females is slightly higher.

7

Hormones begin to influence fetal development at about the seventh week of intra-uterine life. There are three groups of 'sex' hormones and these are:

1   Oestrogens, which predominate in the female
2   Progestins, which predominate in the female
3   Androgens, which predominate in the male

All three types are called 'steroid' hormones because they share a particular type of chemical structure, and they are all produced by the ovary, testis and adrenal glands. Hormonally, females and males differ from each other only in the relative amounts of each type which they manufacture. Ovaries produce mainly oestrogens and progestins, with small amounts of androgen, while testes secrete principally androgens as well as some oestrogen and progestin. The pituitary gland controls the functioning of these other endocrine glands and, because it is situated so close to the brain, is strongly influenced by it.

At about the seventh week of life in utero, then, these hormones come into play and lead to sexual differentiation in the previously 'neutral' embryo. In genetic females ovaries develop, followed by fallopian tubes and a uterus internally, and clitoris, vagina and vulva externally. In genetic males, testes develop and the tubes which would have become fallopian tubes in a female disappear. A different set of tubes appears and one on each side goes on to become the vas deferens. Externally the penis and scrotum develop.

The basic pattern is thus the female one, and if there is no androgen production it is this which will develop further. The active production of androgens is needed to bring about male development. In other mammals the presence or absence of androgens influences brain development, and adults show mainly male or female behaviour as a result (Gray & Drewett 1977). For example, if a genetically female rat is given doses of androgens at birth she will behave sexually more like a male as an adult, being more aggressive and non-receptive to sexual advances by males. However, there is little evidence that hormones have strong effects on the human brain before birth (Money & Ehrhardt 1982).

DIFFERENCES IN INFANCY AND CHILDHOOD

At birth, boys are slightly heavier and longer than girls and these small differences continue, except for a period around eleven years of age when girls overtake boys for about three years because of their earlier onset of puberty. These differences between the sexes are relatively small at all times, and there is more variation among males as a group and among females as a group than there is between females and males (Oakley 1972). This overlap is shown in the illustration of children's weights and heights in Figure 2.1. Hormone levels in girls and boys are also similar until approximately eleven years of age.

More males than females are conceived, but from conception onwards more males than females die at all stages of life, so that there are more females in the population. More male fetuses are

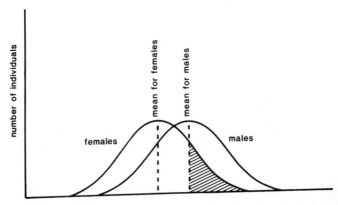

Figure 2.1 Illustration of the normal distribution of weight, height and other variables in women and men. The shaded area illustrates the proportion of female scores which are above the average of male scores

miscarried and more males than females die of birth injuries and congenital malformations. In the first year of life, 54 per cent of all deaths are male and females have a longer life expectancy at all stages. Males appear to be more susceptible to sex-linked genetic diseases and defects, and it may be that one of the female hormones is protective in some way (Bartels 1982). This evidence highlights the fact that claims that men are stronger than women apply to a limited range of evidence, and in many respects it is the male who is weaker and more vulnerable.

PUBERTY

Girls on average reach puberty earlier than boys, although there is a great variation in its age of onset in both sexes and between different cultures and races (Oakley 1972). There is a worldwide trend towards a decrease in the age of starting menstruation, which now occurs on average around the age of twelve. The earlier onset of puberty in girls, with its growth spurt, explains why at certain ages girls are taller than boys of the same age.

Sex hormone action triggers the start of puberty and in girls rising oestrogen levels lead to breast development, a changed distribution of body fat, and an increase in the subcutaneous fat layer. Body hair growth is produced by the adrenal androgens. Oestrogen and progesterone levels begin to fluctuate cyclically and menstruation occurs. In boys, testosterone produces a deepening of the voice, increased muscle development particularly in the neck, chest and shoulders, and changes in body hair distribution. In addition, it causes growth in the skeleton, and increases in heart and lung size, oxygen-carrying capacity of the blood, and ability to neutralise waste products from muscle activity (Tanner 1970; Glucksmann 1974).

These changes contribute to the different shapes we associate with women and men, but there is a wide variation between one individual and another. Amount and distribution of body hair also vary greatly among women and among men. Hormone levels similarly show great variations, so that determination of sex based on hormone levels is impossible and the buccal smear method is needed for this purpose. Cells from the mouth are collected and stained and in females, who have more than one X chromosome, a particular spot of colour called a Barr body can be seen on the slide.

THE MENSTRUAL CYCLE

The menstrual cycle will simply be outlined here because it is described in detail in physiology textbooks. The cycle has five phases, and during the first phase, menstruation, the ovaries produce low levels of hormones and the lining of the uterus is thin. As phase 2 progresses, oestrogen levels rise and this makes the uterine lining thicker. This phase may be termed the 'proliferative' phase and while it goes on the ovum or egg is maturing in the ovary. Phase 3 is ovulation, or shedding of the egg by the ovary leaving a small scar called the corpus luteum. This leads on to phase 4, or the 'secretory' phase, in which the lining of the womb becomes even thicker as a result of the action of both oestrogen and progesterone. In the fifth or pre-menstrual phase, hormone levels are decreasing as the corpus luteum becomes smaller, and then menstruation (phase 1) begins again. Ovulation, the most fertile time in the cycle, occurs approximately 14 days before the onset of menstruation and therefore, when women have longer or shorter cycles than the 'textbook' 28 days, it is the early pre-ovulation phases which are varying in length. Understanding this is vital to those wanting to use 'rhythm' methods to predict when ovulation will occur and conception is most likely, with the aim of either preventing or achieving pregnancy. Some women experience pain at ovulation which is called 'mittelschmerz', meaning 'middle pain', but this is not usually severe and lasts only a couple of hours.

The menstrual cycle is controlled by the pituitary gland, which secretes the gonadotrophic hormones called luteinising hormone and follicle-stimulating hormone (LH and FSH) which stimulate the ovaries. The male pituitary produces parallel hormones which stimulate the testes. Average actual blood loss during menstruation is 30–40 millilitres, or two eggcupsful, but the amount may vary between 10 and 90 millilitres. The quantity appears greater because the uterine lining is shed at the same time. Vaginal secretions also vary with the menstrual cycle, being scanty just after menstruation, becoming much thicker and whiter at ovulation, and perhaps even thicker in the pre-menstrual phase. Some women are able to use these changes as signs of the progress of their cycles and as an aid to judging when ovulation takes place (Birke & Gardner 1979).

PRE-MENSTRUAL TENSION

It has never been scientifically demonstrated that the cyclical hormone changes of menstruation are connected with mood changes. Various theories about the cause of pre-menstrual tension (PMT) or pre-menstrual syndrome (PMS) have been suggested, including attributing it to progesterone deficiency, involvement of adrenal hormones, and high prolactin levels. These ideas point to fluid retention as causing the symptoms, while the vitamin B6 (pyridoxine) deficiency theory claims that steroid hormones alter brain chemistry and cause mood changes (Birke & Gardner 1979).

Dr Katharina Dalton is perhaps the best-known worker in the PMT field, and she has appeared in court on a number of occasions in defence of women who were said to have committed crimes while under the influence of progesterone deficiency and its resulting PMT. She claims to be able to cure PMT by administering doses of progesterone but has not conducted satisfactory double-blind trials, and so a placebo effect cannot be ruled out. In a double-blind trial of progesterone therapy carried out by other researchers, its performance was no better than a placebo. Nor have studies been able to show any systematic difference between the hormone levels of PMS suffers and non-sufferers. Similarly, women with the lowest progesterone levels do not have signi-ficantly different symptoms from others (Laws 1983).

Fashions seem to arise at different periods in history, when 'experts' pick out certain 'symptoms', develop 'scientific' explana-tions for them, and initiate treatments which may be expensive, restrict people's lives, and cause iatrogenic (treatment-induced) complications. Women historians have recently brought to light practices carried out by Victorian doctors which we would consid-er scandalous if they were performed today. Vaguely-defined symptoms which these doctors grouped together as 'woman's troubles' included nymphomania, masturbation, 'eating like a ploughman', 'cussedness', and persecution mania. These 'prob-lems' were attributed at one time to the ovaries, which were thought to control the personality, and many 'ovariectomies' were carried out to remove the supposedly diseased organs and render women 'tractable, orderly and cleanly'. Attempts were made to control the 'wandering womb' of 'hysterical' patients, for example, by placing numerous substances and objects in the vagina, ranging from tea and marshmallow to leeches. Later in the 19th century the rest cure, involving total isolation and sensory de-privation, was prescribed for 'female disorders' (Ehrenreich & English 1979).

Fashions inevitably change with the passage of time. The symp-toms included in PMS, although similarly vague, are different from the 'women's troubles' of the last century and the treatments prescribed are different too. It certainly cannot be denied that some women experience changes in the way their bodies function at various stages of the menstrual cycle, and these may feel unpleasant. But evidence does not prove that hormones are the cause of these problems, and we shall look at alternative inter-pretations in the following chapters on psychological and sociolo-gical theories of sexuality.

ADULT SEXUALITY

Adult females and males in our society have a somewhat different physical appearance and customarily perform different roles in the home and at work outside. How did these differences come about? Charles Darwin's evolutionary theories, built upon by his followers who include Desmond Morris of 'Naked Ape' fame, attempt to explain physical and role differences as adaptations of the human organism to ensure species survival (Morris 1967). The well-known phrase 'survival of the fittest' sums up his idea that only the strongest will survive and weaker, less well-adapted members will be bred out of the species. Darwin's theory of evolution is founded on the proposal that two mechanisms determine which individuals will produce the most offspring to carry on the species. The first of these mechanisms is competition among males for females, and the second is choice by females of males possessing certain characteristics rather than others. Thus males' greater size, strength and aggressiveness have evolved in the competition to win over and impregnate females, who prefer these characteristics in their mates, according to this theory. Female preference has also been given as an explanation for why men developed beards. Correspondingly, female breasts, their rounded body shape and relative absence of body hair are said to have come about by a process of elimination, leaving such females to survive because males find them more sexually attractive. Desmond Morris agrees with the theory that the female body evolved along these lines 'to make sex sexier' for the male and to promote long-term, stable relationships between males and females for the purpose of rearing children. However, it is not necessarily true that increased sexual attractiveness would lead to more stable relationships. It is also possible that sexual attractiveness could be disruptive, with increased competition and choice encouraging more short-term relationships (Birke *et al* 1980).

Alternative, less male-centred interpretations of how women's and men's bodies have evolved see the female shape as an adaptation for giving birth and rearing children. In other mammals, female breasts develop when the animal is pregnant, and not at puberty as in humans. Early breast development in human females may be an adaptation to provide a greater supply of adipose tissue as a food reserve for pregnant and lactating women in times of shortage. This adaptation would then be for the benefit and survival of the woman and her child, and not for sexual stimulation of the males of the species. Similarly, broadening of the female hips over the course of time may have occurred to accommodate the increasing size of the baby's head as the human brain evolved (Archer & Lloyd 1982).

Biological explanations of different roles for women and men are based on the argument that the division of functions in human reproduction forms the essential and unalterable basis for the division of labour between the sexes in other spheres. If women carry unborn children in their bodies, give them birth, and nourish them by breast-feeding in the early stage of life this logically implies, so the argument goes, that they are best suited to caring for and rearing them throughout childhood until they can live independently. This argument is extended to claim that, since women are less mobile because of their child-centred activities, it is also logical that they should remain in the home and provide domestic services for others, whether these are their male partners, other adults, or old people. The 'maternal instinct' which fits them for motherhood also equips them for caring for other adults, but especially for men.

Men, on the other hand, are physically independent with regard to childbirth and lactation and thus are more mobile and not confined to the home. Their greater physical strength equips them to work outside the home, either to hunt animals and provide meat for women and children as they did centuries ago, or to work in factories, offices and external sites as they do today. Early 'hunter-gatherer' societies are seen as the prototype of present-day society, with a 'natural' division of labour based on reproductive functions which inevitably persists today, albeit with refinements, because it is the most suited to human survival.

Analogies with hunter-gatherer societies are based on a very simplistic description of how these societies functioned in the past, and still do today in some parts of the world. The sexual division of labour is by no means as clear-cut as the model implies, with men going out hunting for meat and women cultivating and gathering food. In some tribes, such as the Mbuti pygmies and the Australian aborigines, hunting and gathering are shared equally among women and men, and among the !Kung it is women who go on hunting and foraging expeditions (Oakley 1972). In Western societies up to the industrial revolution families worked together as production units, with women, children and men forming a team to run the home, grow food and manufacture other goods for subsistence and a surplus for sale or exchange. The industrial revolution took manufacturing work away from the home and into factories and, although this led to some decline in paid employment for women, the effect varied between town and country, and between social classes. Today in Britain, 40 per cent of the paid labour force is made up of women and 70 per cent of married women aged between 35 and 54 go out to work, playing an essential role in supporting their families financially as well as being responsible for the majority of housework and childcare (Oakley 1981).

Just as a neat division of work roles is rare, so a relatively clear division of labour in childcare is by no means universal. Arapesh men routinely undertake the daily care of children equally with women and in perhaps the majority of societies, including our own, the time when women devote themselves exclusively to childcare is very short. In rural societies such as the Alor and Yangan, women work in the fields until they are an hour or so from childbirth and they return immediately afterwards, some-times again within a matter of an hour. Among the Dakota and Bororo, women share breastfeeding of all babies, some staying in the camp to do this while others go out to work (Oakley 1972).

Heavy work demanding great physical strength is not done uniquely by men in rural societies, but also by women who cultivate, harvest and carry crops to market without mechanical aids. In our own society, women do heavy manual labour in nursing or other jobs requiring great physical stamina, such as serving in a shop, which involves standing all day and lifting stocks of goods to replenish displays. Housework and childcare are also extremely physically demanding, again involving lifting heavy weights like children, invalids, shopping, furniture and wet washing.

Studies of physical strength, stamina and physique have shown vast differences between various societies and between different classes within single societies. Birth weights and heights vary more within the sexes than between them, as we saw earlier, and food intake and socio-environmental factors can have a greater influence than sex on weight and height (Bartels 1982). Among the Mundugumou of New Guinea, Margaret Mead found that women were as tall as men, and that food was plentiful and shared out until everyone had had enough. In other areas, such as in Nigeria today, almost all children who die of severe malnutrition are females because male children are given preferential treatment at mealtimes.

She says she wants to be a builder when she grows up, but I told her women aren't made for heavy work like that.

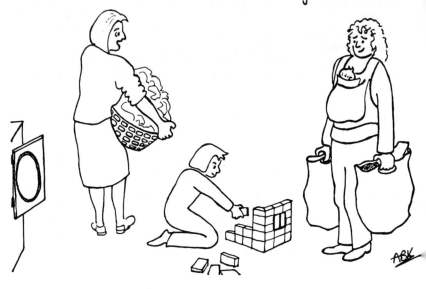

The body physiques accepted in our society as characteristically female and male are not the same as those in other cultures. In the Admiralty Islands women and men have the same physique, with broad shoulders, heavy limb muscles and little subcutaneous fat. These differences may be related to one or more of the factors mentioned already, including ethnicity, diet, life-style and environmental influences. Body shape and muscle strength can also be affected by work and training. Research has shown that women can increase their muscle strength by weight training without altering body shape, and the effect of training of this type is equivalent in women and men. Body shape and strength differences in our own culture may be largely due to the different types and amounts of sports played in childhood. Women have smaller hearts and lungs, but this is partly compensated by higher resting heart rates. Vital capacity of the lungs is smaller and percentage of haemoglobin is lower in females, but these too are alterable by training. Women have a lower systolic blood pressure than men, and one conclusion that could be drawn from this is that they are better physiologically adapted to survive stress (Bartels 1982). Strength differences between women and men are not natural and immutable then, and when some female activities are considered, women's strength and stamina are truly impressive. We only need to think of pregnancy and labour to realise that!

Biological theories of women's and men's greater 'innate' and 'natural' suitability for certain roles in adulthood leave a vast amount of variation still to be explained, and they create the impression that differences between women and men are greater than they are in reality, both with regard to sexuality and physical sex acts.

SEXUAL ACTIVITY

Contradictory attitudes towards sexual activity in both women and men abound in our cultural and religious history. In Christian tradition, women are seen either as madonnas, imitating the pure, virginal image of Mary, or as whores and temptresses like Eve, who lure men into sin and sexual excess. The madonna-like woman is not interested in sex for her own pleasure, but only as a means to motherhood and to gratifying her husband's sexual needs. The whore or Eve-like woman, on the contrary, has an insatiable sexual appetite, seduces men, and is responsible for their downfall and for the sins of the world (Weinberg 1982).

In Victorian times opposing views of women's and men's sexual needs became established, and their legacy is still influential today. Women were seen as having little or no sex drive, and being motivated to endure sexual activity only to satisfy their 'maternal instincts'. Men, however, were said to have enormous and uncontrollable sex drives, and were advised to go to prostitutes in order to satisfy themselves and save their wives from their savage excesses. Inborn biological instincts were seen as the causes of both female and male sexuality (Ehrenreich & English 1979).

Not until the 1930s did systematic study of sexual behaviour begin. Alfred Kinsey and his colleagues in the USA interviewed over 10,000 people between 1938 and 1953 about all aspects of their sex lives. Men reported more sexual activity than women at all ages and, while the frequency of sexual activity for males reached a peak in the early 20s, female activity peaked in the 30–45 age group. The smallest difference in rates between women and men were reported in this latter age group, and it seems that for women marriage was important in influencing frequency of sexual activity

(Kinsey, Pomeroy & Martin 1948; Kinsey, Pomeroy, Martin & Gebhard 1953).

As well as frequency, Kinsey studied the kinds of sexual activity which led to orgasm. Unmarried women reported the highest frequency of masturbation, and 95 per cent of these said they achieved orgasm in this way. For married women, intercourse was the most common source of sexual activity, and 68 per cent of men and 80 per cent of women who had been to university reported having premarital intercourse. Homosexual activity at some time was reported by 25 per cent of males over 15 years old and 3 per cent of females, while 10 per cent of males and 1 per cent of females said they were exclusively homosexual.

Many of Kinsey's findings caused surprise, especially the unexpectedly high levels of masturbation, premarital intercourse, female sexual activity and homosexuality. However, caution is needed in accepting reports by individuals of what they do, because they may underestimate or exaggerate in response to social standards and what they think the interviewer wishes to hear. Therefore their statements do not necessarily accurately reflect their actual behaviour.

These criticisms were avoided by William Masters and Virginia Johnson, who reported in the 1960s on their extensive laboratory studies of sexual arousal and orgasm in women and men. They observed and studied 382 women aged from 18 to 71 and 312 men aged from 21 to 81, and developed a description of sexual response which is divided into four phases, as illustrated in Figure 2.2. The most striking impression is that there is little difference between female and male responses, and Masters & Johnson (1966) were able to explode a number of myths on the basis of their data. Kinsey's finding that women are able to have multiple orgasms following each other within a relatively short time was confirmed, and the clitoris was shown to be the site of sexual excitation, whether stimulation was physical or emotional. A distinctly separate vaginal orgasm was said to be impossible because appropriate nerve endings did not exist in the vagina. In men, it was shown that a large penis did not make for greater female satisfaction, but could cause pain and thereby reduce the woman's pleasure. No correlation was found between the size of the erect and non-erect penis, nor between size of penis and any other organ. 'Withdrawal' was found to be a hazardous contraceptive technique because the majority of men produce a pre-ejaculatory

FEMALES	MALES
EXCITEMENT STAGE	
nipple erection	nipple erection
skin flush	

PLATEAU STAGE

skin flush	skin flush
carpopedal spasm	carpopedal spasm
generalised muscle tension	generalised muscle tension
hyperventilation	hyperventilation
increased heart rate	increased heart rate

ORGASM STAGE

specific muscle contractions	specific muscle contractions
hyperventilation	hyperventilation
increased heart rate	increased heart rate

RESOLUTION STAGE

sweating	sweating
hyperventilation	hyperventilation
increased heart rate	increased heart rate

Figure 2.2 Stages of body responses during sexual arousal described by Masters & Johnson (1965)

fluid containing sperm, and so the woman could be impregnated even if ejaculation did not take place within the vagina. Pregnant couples were studied and it was shown that intercourse did no harm to the unborn child, and research with elderly people demonstrated that they continued to have sexual feelings and the ability to express these. High levels of masturbatory activity in women and men were again reported, as they had been by Kinsey. Masturbatory techniques in women varied greatly according to whether the clitoris was directly stimulated or whether areas such as the mons veneris were the focus. Masters & Johnson therefore suggested that textbook 'recipes' for stimulation during foreplay should be replaced by recommending that couples talk to each other about what gives them pleasure.

Masters & Johnson's research was truly pioneering in the way it described systematically how women and men respond physiologically during sexual activity. This is a limited perspective, however, for sexuality involves so much more than physical acts of sex. There is a great deal more to these physical acts than physiology, and Masters & Johnson's work sheds little light on why people have certain sexual preferences or indeed what brings about sexual attraction and desire between people. Androgens are the hormones associated with sexual arousal in both sexes, but again this is clearly not the whole story. Psychological and sociological factors are what stimulate androgen production and initiate the whole process of attraction and arousal. Biological explanations alone are therefore insufficient for understanding sex acts just as they are for understanding sexuality.

So far, we have discussed sexual activity mainly as a biological event without commenting on the type of activity or partner involved. Whether sexual activity is focussed genitally, orally, anally or on other parts of the body, whether or not penetration occurs, whether there is a partner or not, and if so whether that partner is of the same or different sex, are irrelevant to the purely physiological processes of excitation and orgasm, as Masters & Johnson confirmed.

HOMOSEXUALITY

Homosexuality is still viewed by many people as a deviant minority activity, which is 'unnatural' or sinful and more common in men than women. Kinsey's work posed a fundamental challenge to these ideas, reporting that 37 per cent of white males and 13 per cent of white females in the USA had had actual homosexual experience leading to orgasm at some time in their post-adolescent lives. Kinsey believed that no individual is exclusively either homosexual or heterosexual, and so he devised a 7-point scale ranging from 0 to 6 to describe homosexuality. Those who had never had orgasm with someone of the same sex scored 0, and those with entirely homosexual experience scored 6. Many people who had had varying amounts of heterosexual and homosexual experiences were placed at intermediate points. Kinsey's figures and those of later researchers show that homosexual activity is more widespread than many people believe. Research confirms that homosexuality cannot be considered as a single category, and that behaviour ranges from having genital sexual activity solely with people of the same sex to occasionally experiencing feelings of attraction towards others of the same sex.

Nevertheless, a view of homosexuality as pathological persists in popular culture, and it was as recently as 1973 that the American Psychiatric Association removed homosexuality from its list of diseases. Searches for biological explanations for homosexuality have not been successful. Hormonal theories grew out of observations of animals such as rats, in which insufficient testosterone during development results in 'behavioural feminism', which has been equated with homosexuality. Behavioural feminism means that the animal adopts a passive role in sexual acts whereas homosexuality involves choice of sexual partner, and this 'rato-morphic' or rat-oriented view of human behaviour has proved misleading, for human females exposed to androgens in utero show no greater trend towards homosexuality than controls. In a tiny number of cases, researchers have found lowered testosterone levels in homosexual men and raised levels in women, but in the vast majority of studies no hormonal differences have been found between those whose sexual preference is homosexual and those whose preference is heterosexual (Money & Ehrhardt 1972).

In our culture other kinds of sexual activity may be erroneously labelled as homosexual. Trans-sexuals are people who are genitally of one sex but psychologically of another, and they do not usually have a homosexual preference. Trans-sexuals may seek sex-change treatments and operations to bring their external appearance and internal self-concept to a match. Transvestites are usually heterosexual men who derive pleasure from dressing in the kinds of clothes more commonly worn by women.

In other societies, definitions and norms are very different from our own. Anthropologists' surveys have found that in 49 of the 76 cultures from which the relevant information is available, homosexuality is viewed as normal. This knowledge, together with lack of support for biological theories and awareness of the wide range of sexual expression our own society, must lead to questioning of definitions of homosexuality as a minority, deviant or unnatural activity. An alternative view, which is increasingly although very slowly gaining acceptance, is that homosexual activity is a healthy expression of sexuality and is no different in this respect from heterosexuality, and that condemnation of homosexuality and feelings of guilt and shame are inappropriate.

THE MENOPAUSE

The menopause is another biological event surrounded by much myth and confusion in our culture. In women, the sexual role of oestrogen is restricted to menstruation, ovulation, conception and gestation. Oestrogen does not control sexual drive, erotic thoughts, sexual sensations or ability to have orgasms, and this is a clear difference between human females and some other mammals. After the menopause, when oestrogen falls to minimal levels, women maintain interest and pleasure in sexual activity, and for some desire and satisfaction may be enhanced because fears of pregnancy are gone. In rats, on the other hand, removal of the ovaries leads to disinterest in mating and this example further illustrates the dangers of using animal analogies to explain human behaviour (Archer & Lloyd 1982; Birke *et al* 1982).

Women's reproductive life usually ends between the ages of 45 and 55, when oestrogen levels fall greatly. This transitory period of adjustment may cause dryness of the vagina and urethra, with soreness (atrophic vaginitis) and increased susceptibility to infections, as well as hot flushes. Longer-term changes associated with normal ageing begin at this time too, and include loss of skin elasticity and increased brittleness of the bones due to decreased mineral deposition (osteoporosis), but other supposed menopausal symptoms are a much more complex issue.

Many people associate the 'change of life' with depression, weight gain, and a variety of other symptoms including tiredness, headaches, insomnia and digestive problems, but it has not proved possible to link these with falling hormone levels. Other events in women's lives at around the same time seem more likely causes of mood changes, and children growing up and leaving home, or declining capacity for physical exertion at home and at work can cause anyone to feel 'low' or even depressed at whatever age they occur. Studies have shown that women report more symptoms when they are experiencing these kinds of stressful life events in their early 40s than when their hormone levels are dropping in the early 50s (Greene & Cooke 1980). The proportion of women reporting mood disturbances during the menopause has been found to be 7 per cent, compared with 6 per cent at other times of life, and therefore the size of the problem seems to have been exaggerated. Higher levels of symptoms are reported by middle class housewives who have no fulfilling social role when their families are dispersed, in comparison with those who work outside the home, and symptoms vary between cultures according to whether the society emphasises child-bearing as a defining characteristic of femininity. Where having children is seen as women's most important role, greater distress occurs at the time of the menopause because women suffer a fall in social status. In cultures where old people are accorded high prestige, few such problems are found (Bart 1971). This suggests that hormone changes are not responsible for so-called menopausal symptoms, and the term 'empty nest syndrome' has been coined to describe physical and emotional disturbances of this kind (Hotchner 1980).

In the light of this evidence, the use of hormone replacement therapy (HRT) with oestrogen and/or progesterone to treat menopausal symptoms is questionable in the same way as are hormone treatments for PMT. The symptoms said to be reversed by HRT are usually not severe, last for a year or two at most, and may respond to less dangerous treatments or placebos in some cases. HRT has been implicated in the development of certain types of cancer, and therefore promises of 'eternal femininity' are dearly bought. Vitamin D and calcium supplements may be a safer protection against osteoporosis.

Men have no parallel, relatively rapid end to testosterone production. Testosterone levels decline gradually over the middle to later years, but mood changes and depression may occur around the time of retirement from paid work. We shall follow up this clue to alternative explanations for depression in both women and men in the following chapters.

SEX AND AGEING

Prejudices and misunderstandings pervade our thinking about sex and elderly people perhaps more than any other social groups. Older people are often thought of as sexless, and this is particularly so of post-menopausal women. We have seen that cessation of ovarian activity does not remove sexual desire or capacity, which depend on psychosocial factors and androgen production and not oestrogen and progesterone levels. With men too, sexual activity may be thought to decline with the appearance of other more visible signs of ageing, such as thinning and greying hair and declining physical strength.

In reality, physiological changes play a relatively small part in sexual functioning in the elderly. In women, vaginal lubrication takes longer and may be less in amount, and vaginal expansion and uterine contractions during orgasm are decreased. The labia do not become erect and the pad of fat under the mons veneris becomes smaller. The clitoris changes little, but low oestrogen levels can cause pain on clitoral stimulation, as well as vaginal soreness and uterine spasm during orgasm. Women remain able to have multiple orgasms and their libido can be greater after the menopause, when androgen levels are balanced by low oestrogen levels and the fear of pregnancy is gone (Weg 1983).

Men, when they reach their 60s, take longer to have an erection and the pressure and volume of ejaculatory fluid may decline. While desire for sexual activity may remain, the subjective need for ejaculation itself may be less and erection is lost more rapidly after ejaculation (Weg 1983).

If people are unaware that these physiological changes are normal, men may suffer from performance anxiety and women may feel rejected if their partner does not ejaculate. Contrary to popular belief, sexual activity in older heterosexual couples ceases more often because of male factors than female disinterest. Illness, loss of libido and impotence are some reasons for this, but specialists agree that, as at other times of life, psychosocial factors play a greater role than physiological causes. Cultural prescriptions and proscriptions of what is acceptable behaviour in relation to sexuality, together with lack of knowledge and low levels of communication, feature prominently in people's minds and lead to feelings of guilt, shame and embarrassment (Hendricks & Hendricks 1978, Webb in press).

CONCLUSION

This review of biological aspects of human sexuality throughout the life cycle has shown that, while biology plays a part in explaining how we behave and how we see ourselves as sexual beings, a great deal remains unexplained by this approach alone. Some apparently commonsense biological concepts have not stood up to scrutiny. We saw, for example, that physique can be as much a question of life-style and resources as of genetics, and that what have been thought of as the sexual activities of small minorities are in fact widely encountered throughout all layers of society.

Discussing these questions inevitably involved entering the nature-nurture debate begun by Francis Galton in the last century. Biological determinism is the name given to theories which see biology as the fundamental influence which determines human development and behaviour. An alternative term is biological reductionism, in which explanations are reduced to the biological level in the last analysis. In the next two chapters, we shall see what psychological and sociological thinking can add to our understanding of human sexuality by focussing more on the 'nurture' side of the argument.

CHAPTER 3

Psychology and Sexuality

Some psychologists seeking to account for human sexuality have proposed explanations which, on closer investigation, turn out to be versions of the biological determinism criticised in Chapter 2. They have reduced questions of gender identity and gender roles, or our self-concepts and behaviour as sexual people, to genetic sex and its biological consequences.

Brain lateralisation theory, for example, attempts to explain behaviour differences associated with feminity and masculinity in terms of the control of mental abilities by the right and left halves of the brain. Specialisation of the two cerebral hemispheres exists, the dominant left hemisphere being the site of language processing and the right hemisphere dealing with spatial processing. Women and men have been found to be different in the way this lateralisation functions, males showing earlier specialisation for some spatial tasks. The extent of these differences and their implications for mental ability are questionable, but proponents of the theory have gone on to suggest that the greater numbers of men doing scientific and engineering work, for example, result from brain lateralisation and that this kind of psychological difference is innate. For women, their higher scores on tests of verbal ability are attributed to specialisation of the left hemisphere, where the speech centre is sited (McGee 1979), and are said to equip women better for the verbal communication needed for bringing up children.

Brain size is another factor which has been used to explain why more men than women achieve high levels in educational, work and artistic spheres. The average circumference of male heads is greater than that of female heads, but this is because brain size is correlated with body size, and males are on average larger than females in our society. In fact, the average female has a slightly bigger brain in proportion to her body weight than the male, but head circumference and brain size are not known to be related to intellectual performance (Oakley 1972).

The effect of sex hormones on brain development has also been suggested as a cause of differences in female and male achievements on tests of intellectual ability and temperament, but evidence is weak and hormonal theories have been criticised in Chapter 1.

The social Darwinist analogy with hunter-gatherer societies is the explanation which has gained greatest currency, through popular books by Desmond Morris (1967) and Corinnes Hutt's *Males and Females* (Hutt 1972). Their argument is that women and men have certain psychological traits because these were adaptive for survival and have therefore become fixed in the genetic make-up of the species. Women score higher on tests of verbal ability because this is adaptive for rearing children, communicating with them and teaching them to speak. For men, greater spatial abilities have developed because these are adaptive for hunting. Temperamental differences are explained in the same way, women's roles requiring traits of nurturance, tolerance and emotional sensitivity and men's roles needing more independence, aggression and rationality (Sayers 1979).

The implication of these biologically-based explanations for gender differences is that, if the differences are innate, attempts to change social roles or bring up female and male children in different ways are pointless and doomed to failure. Behavioural and temperamental differences are as they are because humans have certain biological constitutions which have inevitable effects on gender identity and roles. This seems to be a powerful and persuasive argument, but how well does it stand up when evidence on temperamental and intellectual differences is examined?

TEMPERAMENTAL DIFFERENCE

Women and men do behave differently on the whole, as we see for ourselves every day of our lives, and psychologists have attempted to confirm that the sexes differ fundamentally through a number of research strategies. In an early and influential study, Rosenkrantz in 1966 asked university students in the USA to list the attitudes, characteristics and behaviour which they thought distinguished between the personalities of women and men. The items obtained were then arranged in two lists, to represent typically feminine and typically masculine descriptions, and the items on which there was at least 75 per cent agreement between students were selected as representing stereotypes of feminine and masculine personalities. The resulting feminine stereotype suggested that women were more easily influenced, dependent, emotional, excitable, talkative and interested in their appearance, while the male version featured aggression, self-confidence, ambition and objectivity.

These research findings match well the characteristics which Darwinists tell us are the adaptive characteristics of women and men, required for nurturing children on the one hand and for economic survival on the other, but there are a number of problems with the research methods used and these lead to doubt about the conclusions which may justifiably be drawn from Rosenkrantz's study. Firstly, the research set out to study personality differences and the methods used ensured that two lists of different characteristics would emerge. Therefore no other findings than the existence of two different clusters were possible. More recent research into gender stereotypes by Sandra Bem (1974) has shown that people do not conceptualise femininity and masculinity as two opposite extremes. Bem asked students to list their own personality characteristics and then studied whether these conformed to expectations of femininity and masculinity. The findings showed that individuals did not see themselves as having predominantly feminine or masculine attributes, but as being made up of a cluster of mixed characteristics. She concluded that femininity and masculinity were not polar opposites but two distinct concepts, and that some people defined themselves as having approximately equal representations of each. She termed these individuals 'androgynous'.

Another difficulty with gender stereotypes research of this kind results from its reliance on verbal descriptions of difference. Other work suggests that people hold important attitudes which are not easily verbalised and may therefore not be picked up in this way (Sayers 1979).

The view that these stereotypes represent universal attributes of women and men which have evolved to ensure species survival is open to doubt when evidence from other cultures is examined. Anthropologists have found that among the Arapesh people of the Torricelli mountains in New Guinea both women and men are seen as gentle, passive and nurturing, and there are no differential expectations for the sexes. Among the Mundugumou of New Guinea, women and men are equally assertive and independent, while the Tchambuli people of the New Guinea lakes seem to have reversed our expected stereotypes of femininity and masculinity. Thus, all possible combinations of characteristics have been observed, and anthropologists consider that the differences or similarities can always be traced back to different child-rearing practices. In our culture, quite young children have marked preferences for certain toys, boys preferring 'masculine' toys such as wheelbarrows, cars and construction sets and girls choosing 'feminine' toys like dolls' wardrobes and cleaning sets. That these preferences emerge very early does not necessarily indicate that they are inborn, but could equally well suggest that cultural learning begins when we are very young (Oakley 1972).

What conclusions can be drawn from this evidence on temperamental differences between women and men? The only possible interpretation is that the stereotypes reflect commonsense cultural definitions of femininity and masculinity. The mere existence of the differences tells us nothing about their origins, but cross-cultural studies, as well as those of our own culture, suggest that biology does not play a decisive role because temperamental differences are not consistent between societies or even within societies.

INTELLECTUAL DIFFERENCES

Research into a large number of intellectual differences between women and men in the period from 1966 to 1973 has been reviewed and summarised by Maccoby and Jacklin (1974), who found few consistent differences up to the age of puberty except on tests of verbal ability and visual-spatial ability, and even then the differences were small.

On tests of verbal ability, girls score higher at pre-school and early school stages, but boys catch up by the age of ten. Girls remain better at grammar, spelling and verbal fluency throughout school life, however. On general intelligence tests girls also score higher before they go to school, but this gradually reverses with passing time.

Girls learn to count earlier, but as school careers advance boys do better on mathematical tests and this is thought to be due to the greater visual-spatial ability reported by Maccoby and Jacklin. Tests of visual-spatial ability involve making mental transformations in three-dimensional space, as in the example in Figure 3.1. Male advantage on such measures persists into adult life and has been used to account for the larger numbers of males studying and qualifying in subjects like mathematics, physics, engineering and architecture. Maccoby and Jacklin acknowledge that cultural factors can influence scores on these tests because, in cultures where independence is fostered in girls and boys alike, there is no

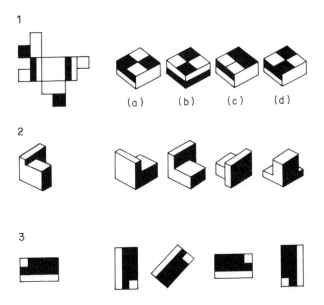

Figure 3.1 An example of psychological tests of spatial ability
In Panel 1, choose which of the four figures labelled A, B, C and D could be made by folding up the object on the left-hand side of the panel.More than one answer may be correct. In Panel 2, choose which of the four objects on the right is the same as the one on the left, just viewed from a different angle. In Panel 3, choose which of the four figures on the right could be produced simply by rotating the left-hand figure. (From *Alice Through the Looking Glass*. 1980. Viragolness Ltd.)

difference in scores. Even where differences are found, the overlap between females and males is similar to those noted in Chapter 1 for weight and height and, although on average males score higher than females, a large proportion of females score above the mean for males.

The study methods used in this type of research can be severely criticised, however, in the same way as those of the temperamental differences research. The first problem arises from the fact that research into intellectual abilities in women and men is again concerned with looking for differences. This means that results showing no differences are ignored and probably not even reported in scientific journals. Secondly, small differences tend to be emphasised at the expense of considerable overlaps in the distribution of test scores (Archer & Lloyd 1982).

Administration of psychological tests is based on assumptions which need to be examined to see whether they are justifiable. Research on the administration of the same test in different conditions demonstrates that scores vary according to the social setting, black children performing differently when researchers are white compared with when they are black, for example (Rosenthal & Jacobson 1968). Anxiety and expectations are just two factors which may influence performance. Also tests may be assumed to measure the same ability when this has not been verified, and some people may use verbal reasoning to complete a test designed to measure visual-spatial ability. Further complications arise when animal tests are compared with human tests, as discussed in Chapter 2. Analogies between visual-spatial ability of rats running through mazes and humans completing pencil and paper tests do not explain why it is valid to assume that the two tests involve comparable intellectual processes.

To understand differences in abilities and achievements between women and men we need to look beyond test scores. It has been estimated that the ratio of women to men in engineering would be 2:3 if entry depended on spatial ability alone, but in fact the ratio is nearer 1:10. To get closer to explaining this, the problem must be approached from another direction by looking at achievement in the context of schooling (Deem 1978; Whitelegg *et al* 1982).

INTELLECTUAL ACHIEVEMENT IN SCHOOLS

Attempts and passes in school examinations reveal a pattern in which at the earlier stages girls achieve more than boys, but in the later stages boys' performance is better. In the days when the 11-plus examination was held, different pass marks were set for boys and girls to ensure equal numbers going on to grammar schools. If the same pass mark had been used for both sexes, there would have been more girls qualifying to enter grammar schools. When CSE (Certificate in Secondary Education), 'O' and 'A' level examinations are considered, slightly more boys than girls enter for no examinations at all, and more boys enter but do not pass. More boys gain CSE passes and more girls gain 'O' levels. Although the differences are small, there is a trend towards better performance by girls on examinations at this level, so that approximately 10 per cent of girls achieve 5 or more 'O' levels, compared with 7 per cent of boys. At 'A' level the position gradually reverses, with slightly more girls getting one or two 'A' level passes, but more boys passing three 'A' levels (Byrne 1978; Deem 1978.

Motivation to achieve seems to be one factor which intervenes to explain this picture. Whereas for boys there is a high correlation between measured IQ (Intelligence Quotient) and school achievement, for girls there is a disparity. In a study of gifted people, IQ and occupational level corresponded closely for men, but two-thirds of women with IQs of 170 or over were housewives or office workers (Oakley 1972). Some external factor therefore influences the conversion of measured ability into achievement in different ways for girls and boys. These differences begin to emerge at a stage in life when girls and boys are being initiated into adult roles. We have seen that achievement and independence for males is culturally valued, while for girls marriage, homemaking and having children are expected and careers are a secondary consideration. The suggestion that girls have learned that academic achievement and femininity do not go together is confirmed by the finding that women college students understate their levels of achievement and pretend to be intellectually inferior to their boyfriends. Boys have been found to attribute academic success to their own abilities, while girls tend to put success down to luck or chance (Deaux 1976). Girls fear failure and are more disturbed by it than boys. Fear of failure and lack of confidence in one's own ability tend to lower achievement in both females and males, but they are found more often in females in our culture (Fransella & Frost 1977).

A great disparity also exists between the subjects studied at school and beyond by girls and boys. Higher percentages of girls study English and foreign languages, religious studies and biology, while more boys than girls take physics, chemistry and mathematics (Byrne 1978; Deem 1978). Girls are more likely to choose science in a single-sex school, and the same is true of boys and languages in boys-only schools. Both sexes have greater access to non-traditional choices in single-sex schools, but there are still wide differences between the subjects taken by girls and boys even in these schools. The differences in single-sex schools have been attributed to the relative absence of different standards for girls and boys and of competition between them, and the fact that in girls' schools science teachers are more likely to be women and to act as role models which endorse science subjects as appropriate for girls. Whatever the reasons, these differences are extremely important because taking certain subjects in particular combinations and at certain levels is crucial for progress into further education and the job market. Pupils who have not studied certain subjects or groups of subjects thereby have their future choices severely curtailed (Curran 1980).

Restriction of some subjects to boys and others to girls is still common (Byrne 1978, Deem 1978). Mixed secondary schools still have separate classes for at least some subjects, and even where 'craft' subjects like woodwork, metalwork, needlework and cookery are open to all pupils, boys are more likely to choose 'girls'' subjects than vice versa. This pattern reflects occupational standards, for men are said to make the best chefs but few women get to the top of the scale in carpentry or engineering. Early specialisation also restricts later choice so that, for example, taking technical drawing at 'O' level may be open only to those who have done metalwork or woodwork earlier. Or choosing biology at 'O' level rather than physics or chemistry precludes going on to a variety of apprenticeship and technological courses.

It is clear that small average differences in verbal and visual-spatial skills between the sexes, even if these exist, are only one factor influencing which subjects pupils study and their levels of achievement. By researching these differences in a way which excludes social factors which operate in real life, inaccurate and irrelevant results are produced and these results then play a part in perpetuating the very differences they claim to have found. Evidence on temperamental and intellectual differences, then, suffers from the defect that the research on which it is based starts off by assuming the existence of certain differences and goes on to claim these same differences as results of the research. Just as we saw with physical attributes, differences in personality and intellectual performance are exaggerated and similarities and overlaps between the sexes are played down.

Psychoanalytic theory is another attempt to explain behavioural differences between the sexes, and we shall now evaluate what these ideas can add to our discussion of sexuality. Freud's psychoanalytic theories are important because they have been very influential in medical thinking and a vast number of other spheres. Many of our 'commonsense' ideas are derived from Freudian writings without our being aware of this. 'Freudian slips' and 'phallic symbols' are two examples of this influence, but many others are so deeply embedded in our culture that their origins have been forgotten. Nevertheless, their influence in everyday life is profound.

PSYCHOANALYSIS AND SEXUALITY

Freud based his theories of the development of sexuality on the anatomical distinctions between the sexes. He believed that anatomical difference led to the development of two different kinds of personality and through psychoanalytic interviews with patients he built up his theory of how this developmental process occurs.

In early life, all children are 'little men' according to Freud. They are unaware of the differences between females and males, and they gain sensual and sexual pleasure from many body areas including the mouth, anus, clitoris or penis. Their sexuality is thus 'polymorphous' or bisexual. At about the age of 5, children realise that the two sexes are anatomically different, and that they as individuals either have or do not have a penis. A girl, discovering that she does not have a penis, blames her mother for this 'castration' and turns from her previous maternal emotional attachment to identify with her father. The girl feels inferior because she lacks a penis and sees identification with her father as a way to gain one. She sees her mother as a rival in her relationship with her father, and jealousy builds up as the girl has fantasies of a sexual relationship with her father. This 'Oedipal' phase is resolved by puberty, when the girl has accepted the passive nature of her sexuality and transferred the site of her sexual pleasure from the clitoris to the vagina in preparation for genital, reproductive sex (Chodorow 1978).

A boy, on learning that he has a penis, develops fantasies of a sexual relationship with his mother. He fears that his father's jealousy will lead to punishment by taking away his penis, amounting to castration. The boy realises that penetration and impregnation of the female are the aims of sexuality, and he transfers his pleasure exclusively to the penis, so that by puberty he too has repressed his bisexuality (Chodorow 1978).

By puberty, when the Oedipus complex is resolved in both sexes, two distinct patterns of sexuality have thus developed. For girls sexuality is passive, focussed on penetration leading to vaginal orgasm, and its aim is motherhood. Wanting a baby is substituted for wanting a penis. Boys develop an active type of sexuality, similarly centred on penetration as a prerequisite to impregnation of women. Personality structure develops in parallel, according to Freud, with women being passive, reticent, needing affection and being less intelligent because their mental activity is centred on the maternal role. Men have more active, independent and aggressive personalities to match their role of initiative and penetration in the sex act. Men's intelligence develops more because it turns to a wider world beyond childbearing. These two personality patterns also reflect for Freud the role of the ovum and sperm in reproduction. The passive ovum stays inside the female body, while the active, independent sperm seeks out the ovum and joins up with it.

In some 'deviant' cases this developmental process goes wrong, however. Some girls fail to repress their bisexuality and do not accept their maternal role, with its vaginal orientation, and the masochistic pleasure which childbirth brings in the Freudian scheme of things. In this case one of two other outcomes is possible, and the girl either becomes a neurotic woman or a homosexual. Boys who have an unsuccessfully resolved Oedipus complex, failing to repress pleasure from other sites than the penis or to take an active sexual role, may also become homosexual (Archer & Lloyd 1982).

Although Freud's thinking has become very widespread, influential and incorporated into everyday ideas, it has been severely criticised both with regard to its scientific validity and its methods of study. Scientific theories are never totally objective because scientists, like all of us, interpret their observations in the light of their own personal views, social backgrounds and personalities. Being scientific entails subjecting these interpretations to rigorous and systematic testing to see whether the interpretation is valid, but critics of Freud say he failed to do this (Brown 1973).

Freud's own personal background was that of a Jew living in Vienna in the late 19th century and, of course, he was a man. Therefore he lived in an atmosphere of strict sexual morality, in a religious context which strongly favoured the male-dominated family and a subservient role for women, for whom having children was highly valued. He constructed his polar opposite notions of mature femininity and masculinity on this basis and, because he restricted his observations to this limited cultural milieu, he failed to realise that this pattern was not universal. We have seen that sexuality is differently expressed in a variety of cultures other than our own. Recent biographies of Freud have brought out features of his personal life which also undoubtedly affected his interpretations. He had a long-standing sexual relationship with his wife's sister Minna, with whom he went away on holidays and spent a great deal of time discussing his work (Gillie 1982). This relationship would have been socially disapproved of at that time and Freud may have projected his own needs for secrecy and repression over this on to his interpretations of what his patients told him. In addition, he was addicted to cocaine and it is now known that some of the dreams he reported as those of his patients were in fact his own dreams or possibly drug-induced hallucinations (Gillie 1981).

More recent research with children has shown that Freud's formulation of the Oedipus complex and its role in the development of sexuality cannot be accurate. It is now known that children have well-developed concepts of femininity and masculinity by as early as two years of age, when they know unambiguously that individuals are women or men, and that certain types of clothing, hair styles, toys and roles are appropriate to each sex. They are usually unaware of genital differences at this stage, and therefore Freud was wrong both in relation to the timing and the origin of the Oedipus complex and the realisation that sexual differences exist (Chodorow 1978). His theory would not be applicable to societies in which clothes are not worn and children are aware of genital difference from a much earlier age than he suggested, nor would it explain how blind children become aware of femininity and masculinity (Kessler & McKenna 1982).

Other criticisms focus on Freud's methods of study and verification of his theories. Popper, a philosopher of science, has said that theories can only be considered scientifically valid if it is theoretically possible to disprove them by observation and testing. Offering positive evidence by itself is not enough, because it is never certain that, with further research, a contradictory finding would not occur. If a theory stands up to attempts to disprove it, then the probability of its being accurate is increased. A problem with Freud's theories is that they are set out in such a way that they can never be disproved, as the example of the 'double-bind' of femininity illustrates. We saw earlier that maturity in women is defined by Freud as acceptance of a passive sexual role which has as its aims penetration by the penis and motherhood. Freud says that all women have this instinct for motherhood and that this is proved by the fact that they do accept this kind of sexuality. Those who do not have children still have a maternal instinct, but they are repressing it and denying themselves the masochistic pleasure of childbirth (Deutsch 1945). Thus all women are said to have a maternal instinct, whether they demonstrate it or not, and there is no way of disproving its existence because those who do not have children are simply repressing or denying their femininity. We have also seen that empirical testing by Masters & Johnson has refuted a number of basic Freudian concepts including the passivity of female sexuality and the vaginal nature of the female orgasm.

Methodological problems also arise from the fact that Freud's theories are based on observations of disturbed people who came to him for treatment of their problems. It is risky to base definitions of normal personality and sexuality on observations of 'abnormal' or 'problem' cases. Freud has also admitted that his theories of female sexuality were speculative because he understood relatively little about women. Furthermore, his patients were mainly adults and he did little work with children, so his data on childhood sexuality comes from adults' reconstructions of what happened many years before when they were children. The scope for distortion and re-interpretation in their accounts is obvious.

A possible rejoinder to these criticisms might be that what is important is not detailed accuracy of the theories but whether they work. If psychoanalysis helps people who have emotional problems, it might be justifiable even if its finer points are questionable. In 1950 the psychologist Hans Eysenck conducted a study of the efficacy of psychoanalysis compared with psychotherapy and with no treatment for neurotic patients. Forty-four per cent of the psychoanalytically-treated patients improved, as did 64 per cent of the psychotherapy patients. However, 72 per cent of those receiving no treatment at all improved. Many later studies have come up with similar findings, showing that psychoanalysis compares unfavourably with other treatments and that many patients get better in time with no treatment (Brown 1973).

Certain features of psychoanalytic treatment are also worth noting. Theoretically, the psychoanalytic relationship between analyst and analysand (patient) is one of equality, so that analysands will feel completely free and at ease in talking about whatever personal matters they wish to raise. In reality, this can never be so because patients come to the analyst's office and pay for the treatment, which immediately puts the analyst in a 'superior' position, as does the 'expertise' possessed. Even in a public health service setting where no direct payment is made, the relationship is far from equal. Crucially for our discussion, a further inequality arises because in the majority of cases the analyst is a man and the analysand is a woman. Therefore unequal power relations between the sexes from outside the analytic encounter influence what goes on during treatment.

Freudian theory is quite clear in stating that masculinity is the superior and dominant form of sexuality. Females are said to envy males their penises, but males do not envy vaginas. Critics have pointed out that what women actually envy in men is not their penises but what goes along with having a penis, such as social status, more independence in life and a wider choice of interesting, creative and demanding roles. Objectively it is better to be a male in our society, they say (Archer & Lloyd 1982).

We have explored and criticised psychoanalytic ideas about sexuality at some length because they have become very influential in our culture. Despite the criticisms, it must be acknowledged that Freud's work has had some positive influence on our understanding of sexuality. His realisation of the importance of sexuality in all aspects of life was revolutionary at the time and his work has stimulated a wealth of subsequent study. In that sense his ideas were potentially liberating , as was his realisation of the role of the 'talking cure' in treating emotional problems. Unfortunately, due to biases resulting from his personal background, views and philosophy of life, this liberating potential has not been achieved. Stereotypes of appropriate behaviour for women and men have been given a 'scientific' credence which is not justified on the basis of Freud's methods of study, and these stereotypes have been little short of disastrous for some people's concepts of sexuality and health, as we shall see in later chapters. These harmful effects are related also to the implication of Freud's theory that the source of problems in the area of sexuality is in individual people's heads and not in the way society is organised. Individuals are blamed for their own or other people's problems and mothers are condemned for their children's difficulties in life. Finally, we have seen that psychoanalysis is another form of biological determinism, which sees our destiny as a matter of anatomy and innate instincts.

To follow up the undesirable consequences of these ideas for health and sexuality, we shall look in more detail at two Freudian concepts – one affecting women and the other affecting men. These are the maternal 'instinct' and the aggressive 'instinct'.

A MATERNAL INSTINCT?

Wanting a baby is a natural and normal feminine instinct which all women are born with, according to biologically-oriented explanations of sexuality including psychoanalytic theories. In practice things are not so straightforward, as Sally MacIntyre (1976) found in her study of single mothers. As these pregnant women progressed through the medical system either to give birth or to have an abortion, doctors' and nurses' reactions conveyed their beliefs that a maternal instinct was normal and expected only in married women. Single women were expected to want an abortion and were thought peculiar if they did not. Doctors judged keeping the baby as normal if single women intended to get married, but not if they were to stay single. When single women grieved over a miscarriage and refused contraceptive advice because they intended to try to become pregnant again, nurses expressed surprise and thought them abnormal. The view seemed to be that married women had a maternal instinct but single women did not.

Belief in a maternal instinct and a desire to have babies would lead us to expect pregnant women to be contented with their state and to view it as natural. However, a study of symptoms in pregnancy has shown that women who assess themselves as more feminine, expressed in terms such as gentle, emotional and dependent, report more psychiatric symptoms in pregnancy compared with those who see themselves as more 'masculine', strong and self-confident. This suggests a clash between 'feminine' characteristics and being pregnant. Another study has shown that pregnant women undergo a great deal of anxiety over the contradictory expectations associated with femininity. An aspect of ideal femininity is physical attractiveness, but during pregnancy and after delivery women felt unattractive because of their altered shape, stretch marks, and the fact that they could not wear the kinds of clothes they liked. Resentment followed this perceived loss of attractiveness after the birth too, when women felt older, permanently disfigured by physical changes, and demoted in social status if they became full-time housewives (Moyes 1976).

Ann Oakley's research with pregnant women and early mothers shows that women's own expectations of a maternal instinct are not fulfilled (Oakley 1979). Sixty per cent of women interviewed believed in a maternal instinct before the birth but less than half did so afterwards, and the majority were shocked by their lack of maternal feelings after the baby was born. One woman in late pregnancy said

> "It's amazing how boring pregnancy is... I expected to feel much more maternal... but it's just not *me*. I expected – strangely – to undergo some change and have these maternal feelings... I haven't."

Women expected that they would know instinctively how to handle and care for the baby, as some animals do, but they were horrified not only at their inability but also at their feelings of rejection of the baby. One woman said

> "When they first gave him to me I thought 'God, what do I do with this?'"

and another told the researcher

> "I didn't know what the ... to do. There was this kid crying in the cot and I just sort of sat there and then started rocking the cot – shut up, shut up".

Another way in which women did not automatically accept and adjust to their babies focussed on the sex of the child. Only 22 per cent wanted a girl, compared with 54 per cent wanting a boy and 25 per cent not having a particular preference. When they had a boy 93 per cent were pleased, but only 56 per cent were pleased to have a girl. Having a boy was thus almost always pleasing, but approximately half of those having a girl were disappointed.

Having maternal feelings is by no means as automatic for women as it would be if their origins were instinctual. Conversely, it is not only genetic females who enjoy and are good at bringing up children. Obviously many men enjoy childcare and regret that stereotypes and role divisions prevent them taking a greater part in the lives of their own and other people's children. They realise that they are missing many deeply fulfilling experiences in family and working life. Males with chromosome abnormalities who are reared as females, and Turner's syndrome females who have only one X chromosome and are therefore infertile, show nurturing behaviour and are just as adequate at childcare as other people, which again calls into question the genetic or hormonal origins of 'maternal' behaviour (Archer & Lloyd 1982).

In the last analysis, lactation is the only biological factor which binds women to their offspring, and if this were not so 'experts' would not need to write so many books telling women how to be good mothers. The existence of these books teaching motherhood amounts to an acknowledgement that there is no such thing as the maternal instinct, and the tone of some of them seeks to create a romanticised image of mothering which implies that women need to be persuaded to do what is supposed to come naturally. Sheila Kitzinger (1962) for example, writes:

> "The woman feels as if her whole body is becoming a gateway into the world for her child. The head begins to ooze out... The gates swing back and open wide... He suddenly turns red, and the mother gasps with pleasure... She wants to take him into her arms immediately, to hold him tight and soothe him... Whether boy or girl she realises that this child is exactly what she desired."

The women interviewed by Ann Oakley were far from agreeing with this idealised picture and what they said, together with many other research findings, makes the existence of a biologically-based psychological instinct for maternity difficult to accept.

MASCULINE AGGRESSION

Aggression is a personality trait which forms part of our cultural stereotype of expected male behaviour, as we saw in Chapter 2 when considering temperamental differences between the sexes. Some explanations of its origins focus on the possible developmental effects of testosterone on the male brain, but no study has been able to demonstrate how this link might work, nor that it does in fact exist (Archer & Lloyd 1982).

Another theory rests on the now familiar analogy with hunter-gatherer societies, but we have questioned the notion that male aggression is universal by citing intercultural differences in definitions of feminine and masculine behaviour (Oakley 1973). It should also be noted that the concept relies on a particular definition of aggression, ignoring another aspect of gender stereotypes which claims that women show more verbal aggression than men. However, recent research has countered this last claim by showing that, when tape-recordings of conversations are analysed, men are more verbally aggressive in that they speak louder, interrupt more often, and take up a higher percentage of the conversation (Spender 1980).

Despite these confusions and contradictions, male aggression is socially valued and boys show this kind of behaviour at an early age. Early age of onset does not necessarily suggest a biological origin, but can also indicate that learning such behaviour begins very early. Parents expect boys to be more aggressive and so tolerate more of this behaviour, and encourage boys to fight back when attacked by another child. Crying and other 'cissy' behaviour is discouraged in boys, so that among nursery school children boys are more aggressive to other children, more negative towards adults, and more physically active and antisocial compared with girls. Girls are allowed fewer demonstrations of aggression, are discouraged from fighting, kept closer to their mothers, and criticised for 'tomboy' behaviour (Oakley 1972). Therefore it is clear that, even if a biological basis for temperamental differences could be established, learning experiences and differential rewards and punishments would still have a powerful influence.

There is a significant correlation between body size and aggression and, because males are on average larger than females, this could account in part for their greater aggressiveness because large females too are more aggressive than smaller ones (Steinmetz 1977). These behavioural differences are revealed in different crime rates for women and men. Men commit more crimes involving violence, and the numbers of women convicted for malicious damage, robbery (as distinct from larceny or petty theft), housebreaking and sex offences is minute compared with male statistics. Men are also more aggressive towards themselves, as their comparatively high suicide and alcoholic illness rates show. It is difficult to assess crime rates, however, because statistics reflect the use of different categorisations for female and male crimes, and greater leniency in sentencing women in accordance with conceptions of femininity and masculinity. For example shoplifting is more common in women and this may be related to their social role in making purchases for the family, while men steal more cars, which is probably linked to the fact that more men

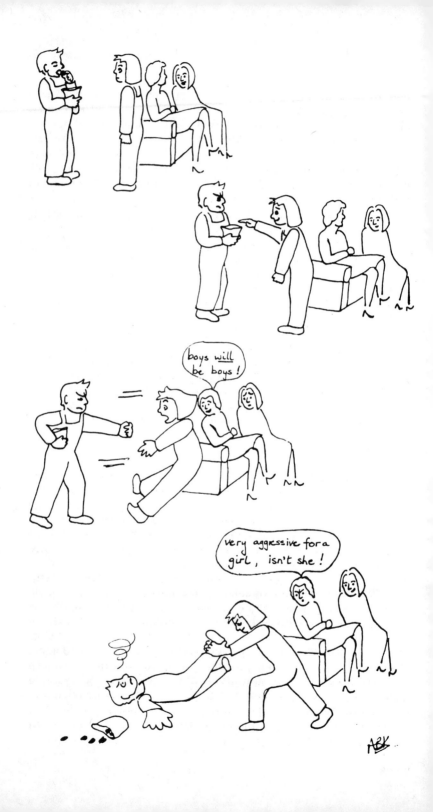

can drive and have learned some car mechanics. 'Women's crimes' are less likely to attract a prison sentence than 'men's crimes', and once in prison the two sexes are treated differently (Hutter & Williams 1981; Oakley 1982).

An extreme expression of male violence and aggression is rape. Commonly-held beliefs about rape are that it is either a spontaneous attack on a stranger, involving uncontrollable sexual urges on the part of the man, or that rapists are mentally sick, sadistic psychopaths. These myths hide a reality in which the majority of rapes are committed by men known to the women concerned, whether as relatives, neighbours or work colleagues, and approximately 50 per cent of rapes take place in the victims' homes. A woman may let the man in because she knows him, or he may break in, perhaps to burgle the house. Over 70 per cent of rapes are planned in advance, as studies have repeatedly shown, and in the region of 50 per cent are pair or gang rapes (Brownmiller 1975). Women frequently report that, far from exhibiting uncontrollable sexual needs, rapists often have difficulty in getting an erection and do not appear to experience much pleasure from the act. Rape seems to be an attempt to exercise power over women, to demonstrate 'virility', or to prove oneself to companions. Some rapists say that they choose to attack women who do not conform in some way, such as by walking alone after dark, living alone, or being a prostitute.

A 'masculine mystique' parallel to the feminine mystique described by Betty Friedan (1963) has been proposed by Diana Russell (1982). According to this idea, rape is an extreme acting out of qualities that are defined as supermasculine in our society. Men feel the need to demonstrate their masculinity by a show of aggression, force, strength, dominance and competitiveness, and this felt need may be greater in men who feel powerless in other areas of their lives. A certain degree of social approval of this kind of acting out is evidenced when films glorifying rape win wide popular acclaim, as did *The Clockwork Orange* and *Coming Home*, and when mass rape in war is condoned.

In recent years, reports of violence and aggression by men have been increasing, but a greater number of reports of rape, incest and wife-beating does not necessarily mean that their actual incidence is rising. It may reflect a greater willingness by women to report offences, different ways of collecting statistics, and different approaches to supporting victims. Rape crisis counselling services and organisations offering refuge to abused women and their children have grown in numbers in recent years as part of the women's movement and they have done much to publicise what was formerly a hidden, 'private' or 'domestic' problem.

The 'masculine mystique' is linked to expectations that men will separate their emotional needs for love and affection from other activities, notably sexual acts, and underplay their caring side. This, together with our culture's emphasis on genital sexuality at the expense of other aspects, enables men to see women as existing for male sexual gratification. As Norman Mailer said, 'It's better to rape than to masturbate'. Cultural definitions of masculinity and femininity, not psychological traits or biological needs, predispose men to rape. They produce a situation where all men are potential rapists and all women are in fear of rape. Until this is understood, ineffective hormone treatments will continue to be given to sex offenders, women will walk in fear, and men will remain emotionally stunted and condemned to act out their fantasies in violence against others and against themselves.

CONCLUSION

In this chapter we have discussed psychological studies of sexuality and found that they usually turn out to be further examples of the biological reductionism noted in Chapter 1. This applies also to psychoanalytic theories, and in many cases methodological inadequacies call the validity of the findings into question.

Social psychologists, however, realise that greater understanding of personality and intellectual achievement cannot be reached unless investigations are broadened to include the social context in which temperament and abilities develop. Social learning theorists have described this learning process as one of imitation, involving rewards and punishments to reinforce or suppress behaviour. Others, the cognitive development theorists, see this as a very passive view of human beings and instead they describe human development as a process of interaction between individuals and their environment, a process in which each can influence the other. In the next chapter we shall focus on these social influences in order to gain a deeper understanding of human sexuality in health and illness.

CHAPTER 4

Sociology and Sexuality

Humans are social beings, whatever their genetic make-up. From the moment of our birth other people respond to us in myriad ways which they themselves have learned, and it is these social influences which make us who we are. We are, of course, born biologically different from each other, but how we view ourselves and how others react to us as sexual beings is something we learn. There is evidence that social factors have effects even before birth, for a pregnant woman's life-style – standard of living, diet, smoking habits and alcohol consumption – influence how a fetus grows and develops, which in turn affect its survival chances in the perinatal period (Oakley 1984). Male life-style factors may have a similar influence.

'Role' is a sociological concept often used to discuss social learning, but it is not altogether satisfactory because it suggests a passive process of socialisation. The analogy linking social roles with roles in the theatre implies that people are cast in roles, learn their lines and follow a script without deviating from it. A closer analogy is that of a game like hockey, where players know the rules, where they can or cannot go on the field, who they may tackle and pass the ball to, how the game is won or lost, and what are the penalties for breaking the rules. They can then choose how to play and can take decisions about what they will do, knowing what the results are likely to be. Although this analogy is closer it still does not completely match social life, because players in a game cannot change the rules, the size or shape of the pitch, or the number of players. In life, by contrast, we interact with our social and physical environments and we can change and be changed by them. We are active agents rather than simply responding passively to cues, rewards and punishments or being 'socialised'.

This 'interactionist' approach involves taking into account how people make decisions about what to do and how to behave as they interact with other social beings. The meanings of situations to the people involved are crucial for understanding how social life goes on. At the same time, we are clearly not free to choose from an infinity of options. Social arrangements already exist when we are born, and these social structures have strong influences on the choices available. The social class system, cultural definitions of gender and the sexual division of labour are some of these social structures within which we live our lives. They influence what choices are available and the results of these choices.

In this chapter we shall focus on social aspects of sexuality. Gender roles will be the main concern, and we shall discuss how we learn to see ourselves as gendered beings, how others react to our sexuality, how we live out our gender roles, and some effects of gender on health. The majority of us learn these first lessons in a family, and this is where we shall begin the discussion.

WHAT FAMILY?

Sociologists have spent much time and energy discussing the family, whether it is a universal institution which exists in every society, and what are its functions. Recently attention has also turned to whether the family is disappearing or being stripped of its functions, which are usurped by schools and social welfare institutions.

Anthropologists have argued that some kind of family unit exists in every society studied, but we have already considered enough evidence in Chapters 2 and 3 to see that, whatever does exist, it is not one universal type of family made up of a married woman and man with their offspring, with or without other additional persons. This 'nuclear' family does not exist in situations where women or men take more than one sexual partner and/or live in an extended family. The nuclear family, comprising a married couple and their joint offspring, is not even the principal family form in our own society. Only 30 per cent of families are made up in this way, and 10 per cent of children are born into single parent families (Oakley 1982). Other 'families' consist of single people, couples of the same or different sex with or without children, and larger groups of people related or unrelated to each other by birth. *The* family, then, is rather hard to locate.

The functions of this unit too are fulfilled in a variety of ways. The sexual function of families clearly may be performed elsewhere, both before and outside marriage where this is practised. The reproductive function similarly does not depend on any particular family form, and 'illegitimacy' is socially defined. In some societies women must become pregnant to demonstrate their fertility before marriage, and reproduction can now take place even in test tubes. The economic function of the family is carried out in enormously varied ways, even within our own society, and increasingly women go into paid employment, making up 40 per cent of the labour force today. Only 1 in 10 households has a sole male breadwinner and a woman full-time housewife (Oakley 1981). Other educational institutions beyond the family share its socialising function, and these include all kinds of communication media such as magazines, newspapers, television and radio.

Families exist in a variety of forms and social functions are fulfilled in numerous ways, so that to talk of *the* family is inaccurate and hides a great diversity. As well as having functions, however, the 'ideal' nuclear family also has dysfunctions. This haven of retreat from the pressures of competitive social life can be a constricting, hostile social grouping and have unequal benefits and costs for its various members. Nevertheless, some form of family remains the place where most children begin to learn their social roles.

LEARNING GENDER ROLES

A baby's sex is probably the first thing that is remarked on at most births and the exclamation 'It's a boy!' is more often a reason for joy and congratulations than 'It's a girl!'. Reports of this in Ann Oakley's study of mothers' reactions to the sex of their babies are not unique (Oakley 1979) and in China, for example, where couples are strongly encouraged to restrict themselves to one child, infanticide of female babies is said to occur. Boys are socially so much more preferred that people kill girls so that they can try again and hope for the desired male next time.

Such strong feelings towards babies of different sexes are very likely to affect parents' responses to their offspring, even if these reactions are not consciously and deliberately different. Research has shown that mothers of newborn babies hold boys for longer in each 24 hour period, and stimulate them more than girls both by touch and eye contact (Parke 1979). Their responses to girls are more often a repetition of the babies' noises and actions. These different reinforcements of behaviour may be the beginnings of different learning of verbal skills and assertiveness discussed in Chapter 3.

Mothers 'fuss' more with girls than with boys, and boys are therefore more autonomous from a very early age. More attention is paid to girls' hair and dress, and boys are more often left alone and allowed to be untidy (Moss 1970). Different types of clothing, particularly with regard to colour and elaborateness, are used soon after birth and the first article put on a baby in a maternity hospital may well be a pink name band for a girl or a blue one for a boy. Fathers play and talk more with boy children, but both men and women look at and play more with babies of their own sex (Parke 1979).

Different toys are provided for girls and boys, so that they begin to play with objects which will later be associated with expected gender roles. Parents provide dolls and flowery decorations in girls' bedrooms, but toy animals and vehicles feature in boys' bedrooms (Rheingold & Cooke 1975). When children are given free choice in an experimental playroom, however, girls and boys spend equal amounts of time with 'masculine', 'active' toys such as big trucks. Opportunities to play with a wide range of toys are restricted in homes but when a choice is available children do not necessarily play with 'gender appropriate' toys.

Girls are kept closer to their mothers, while boys are encouraged to play independently. A female role model is usually much more available to girls, who thereby have greater exposure to traditional female activities and domestic roles (Chodorow 1978), whereas boys have to rely more on older boys and the media for role models because fathers are less accessible. Jobs given even to 5 year olds match expected adult roles, girls being set to laying tables and washing up while boys empty rubbish bins (Newson et al 1978).

Both girls and boys identify more closely with the 'strongest' parent, who controls resources and/or shows more affection. If mothers work outside the home, and thus have greater financial influence than housewives, their girl children tend to be less traditionally feminine and more independent, while their sons are more dependent and likely to seek emotional support from adults (Oakley 1972). Since women tend to be more emotionally demonstrative, both girls and boys are more likely to learn this kind of behaviour from their mothers, but boys learn masculine gender roles more easily from affectionate fathers and male juvenile delinquency is associated with 'paternal deprivation' (Biller 1976). Different kinds of punishments may also be used for girls and boys, with fathers more often using physical punishment on boys and thereby providing a role model for aggression (Fagot 1977).

Nancy Chodorow (1978) is a psychoanalyst who has tried to link this approach with a sociological explanation of how children learn gender roles. She rejects many of the Freudian ideas which were criticised in Chapter 3, including the anatomical basis of the Oedipus complex and a definition of women's sexuality as passive. She focusses on social relations between women, men and children and how these lead to the formation of mental pictures of appropriate gender roles.

Girls and boys begin life in close association with their mothers and their first love and affection comes from a woman. What Chodorow tries to explain is how boys, who are brought up mainly by women, develop masculine gender identities while girls, who are socially disadvantaged in the female role, continue to 'mother' and to reproduce these inequalities. She identifies the imbalance in the division of labour between women and men as the source of personality differences. In the Oedipal phase boys have little experience of males with which to identify, because their fathers go out to work and spend relatively little time with them in the home. Therefore boys come to think of masculinity as the opposite of the feminine role model which they know so well. Masculinity is all that femininity is not, and this masculine 'otherness' is idealised, males being seen as independent, unemotional, self-contained and having roles predominantly beyond the home and childrearing.

Girls, despite the Oedipal phase and identification with the father, continue to be physically close to their mothers and to identify with them for much longer than boys do. They therefore develop qualities of empathy and sharing feelings and, through this continuity of relationships, see themselves as less separate from others. Girls do not turn from their mothers to their fathers, according to Chodorow, but add their fathers to their existing maternal relationships.

This different resolution of the Oedipus complex in girls and boys is the basis for the continuation of mothering by women and the reproduction of gender roles from generation to generation, in Chodorow's view. From this it follows that changes in ways of bringing up children would lead to the development of different kinds of personalities in females and males. If both women and men parented, instead of the present predominance of women's mothering, children's concepts of gender would be entirely different and it is impossible to predict what the effects might be. Role models would be so different that the results might not even resemble what we currently think of as femininity and masculinity. Even Sandra Bem's (1974) concept of androgynous people who have a mix of feminine and masculine characteristics would be too limiting.

This is a tantalising and provocative idea. We have already discussed how differences like a mother going out to work can influence children's notions of gender roles in our own society, and how different social arrangements in other cultures are associated with different personality characteristics. If different kinds of parenting could lead to greater achievement of personal potential in women and more emotional expression in men, these ideas are worth considering. On the other hand, when we come to see the effects of a home-centred role on women's health later in this chapter we may wonder whether yet other social arrangements might not be possible, for confinement to the home would probably lead to detrimental effects for men too.

HOME AS A HAVEN

The decisive effect of the industrial revolution on family life is often seen as the separation of work and home, with the home becoming a haven of rest and refuge from the rigours of economic necessity and the struggle to make a living in factories and offices, with their competitive atmosphere and exhausting work routines. But this picture presents a one-sided view, because even when women work outside the home they still usually do a second or 'double' shift of housework on top of their paid job.

Housework has only recently been taken up as a topic for study and compared with other kinds of work, rather than being classed as non-work because it is unpaid. Oakley (1981) compared women's experiences of housework with men's reports of car assembly and other factory work, which is notoriously monotonous, repetitive and alienating in that people have no control over tasks and the speed of their work (Goldthorpe *et al* 1968). Mechanical, repetitious jobs like ironing were most disliked by women, who preferred more creative activities such as cooking. They saw housework as a series of unconnected tasks which never came to an end, and there was no separation of work and leisure for full- or part-time housewives as there is for men. As soon as the dishes are washed, another meal has to be prepared and more washing up is produced, and the average working week for housewives is 77 hours long.

Men's participation in housework varies little whether women work outside the home part-time, full-time or not at all, and when men are interviewed they tend to over-estimate the amount of housework they actually do. When men do housework both they and women describe their contribution as 'help', implying that it is the woman's main responsibility, and statistics of the amount of this 'help' by no means justify the belief that the division of labour in the home is becoming more symmetrical (Young & Willmott 1973). Increased technology and 'labour-saving' machinery in the home have not meant that housework is reduced for women, because jobs formerly done by men may fall to women when they become 'lighter'. For example, in homes with dishwashers men tend to do less washing up, and disposal of rubbish becomes a woman's responsibility when there is a garbage disposal unit. In addition, the time and labour saved by machines tends to be taken up with more elaborate work, such as cooking more complicated meals in microwave ovens or doing washing in separate batches on different washing machine 'programmes' instead of one big batch of laundry. A further problem is that women and men often have different standards for housework and when men 'help' they do not reach women's expected standards, so their contribution is not seen as satisfactory.

Childcare in the family is fraught with similar problems. Men may only be available to do the more pleasurable and lighter tasks during the week, such as bathing and reading a story at bed-time, and this leads to their exclusion from other routines even when they are present because they have not learned how to do the jobs. It is still a matter of surprise if a man changes a dirty nappy, for example. Women care for children on an unquestioned, regular basis but if a woman goes out one evening the father may 'babysit'. The term 'babysitting' is never applied to women looking after their own children, but fathers' childcare is placed on a par with non-parental child-minding. These different social expectations of women's and men's childcare roles are reinforced in single parenthood, which is far more common for women. Single fathers are thought of as having very special attributes and their unusualness makes it much easier for them to get social welfare provisions like home-helps and nursery places.

Freedom to plan one's own work and the absence of a boss or supervisor are said to make the housewife role preferable to work outside the home, but this is not how women themselves experience their situation. They say they are dominated by a rigid timetable which restricts when and how fast jobs are done, and breaks up their day. Children and husband must be got up and off to work or school, meals and clean clothes must be ready on time, and ferrying back and forth between school or station and home, or to leisure activities, have to be fitted in. Personal time for washing hair, having a bath alone, or going to the doctor or dentist can be very difficult to arrange in this intensive and virtually unchangeable timetable.

Isolation is a heavy disadvantage for full-time housewives, and wanting company and the chance of adult conversation are reasons why women may prefer to have an outside job (Hobson 1978). Even men working in alienating jobs have a chance to meet others and have conversations at break-times to relieve stress and monotony.

These differences in family and married life for women and men are associated with different patterns of mental health, even to the point that 'being a housewife can drive women mad' (Barrett & McIntosh 1982). Wives tend to modify their personalities and life expectations to fit with their husbands' jobs and personal wishes, and suffer loss of self-esteem and control as a result, so that married women have a higher incidence of depression than men. Men have dissatisfactions with marriage in the early years, but are happier when they have been married longer, whereas women become increasingly dissatisfied the longer they are married. Women are more healthy when they live alone, but men have better health when they are married, which suggests that marriage has different costs and benefits according to gender (Gove & Tudor 1972, Williams 1977). The fact that women who work outside the home have fewer depressive illnesses than full-time housewives tends to confirm this interpretation. When men take up a full-time home-centred and childcaring role they report similar feelings of isolation, boredom, strain and lack of self-esteem. Men who lose their jobs also have higher levels of depression than women (Gore 1978), and so simple role-reversal between women and men is unlikely to alleviate these dissatisfactions and related health problems.

Pointing out the disadvantages and restrictions of a home-centred existence must not prevent the recognition that family and home are vital and rewarding aspects of social life. It is the lack of balance for women and men which means that neither can derive the potential pleasure and rewards which they might if things were organised differently. Men often report that outside work interferes with their family life and leisure pursuits, and find that taking care of their children can bring emotional satisfactions they have never previously experienced (Oakley 1981).

VIOLENCE IN THE FAMILY

Learning to be a woman or a man in our culture leads to different role expectations and beliefs about what are appropriate responses in certain situations. Male breadwinners may see the fact that they make all or a major part of the financial contribution to the home as giving them rights to services like prompt meals, clean laundry and their wives' sexual services. These beliefs are buttressed by laws which treat wives' earnings as husband's property and do not recognise the possibility of rape within marriage, and by the reluctance of police to intervene in 'domestic' disputes involving violence to women (Hutter & Williams 1980). Men's economic control over women puts strains on couples' relationships and the fact that men are usually physically stronger means that if a quarrel breaks out women are at a disadvantage.

Tolerance of violence towards women in Western culture, based on beliefs about men's rights to ownership and control of their wives, is evidenced not only in legal practices but also in the way medical services respond. A study of wife-battering has revealed how doctors collude and deny the real cause of women's injuries, which in turn encourages repetitions of the battering. A typical 'career' of a battered woman was reconstructed by examining the case notes of over 400 women in a large hospital in the USA (Stark *et al* 1979). These showed that, when a woman came for treatment giving a story that did not fit the injury, doctors did not question this although they recognised the discrepancy between the injury and the story. After symptomatic treatment the woman was simply returned home to the very setting where the injuries had occurred, and over a period of years she presented herself at the hospital on numerous occasions, usually with increasingly severe injuries each time. As her battering 'career' advanced she visited the hospital because of alcoholism, drug abuse, depression or suicide attempts and instead of 'having' a problem she 'was' a problem. Finally she was reduced to a state where doctors felt they could understand why her husband beat her, because of her 'neurotic', 'hysterical' or 'hypochondriacal' behaviour. Doctors had played a role in maintaining the violent situation by ignoring it and returning the woman to the home, despite multiple hospital attendances which could be seen as attempts to get help and make visible the private battering situation, and by this process the woman was transformed from a victim to a problem.

Men's 'trained incapacity' to share their emotions and their greater learned aggressiveness may tip the balance towards a violent outcome in domestic arguments. In addition, expectations that men will be ambitious and successful at work may lead to 'failure' being taken out on those who are less able to defend themselves, a situation which exists hidden from public view in the home. Violence can then be seen as the culmination of a number of social factors, and this interpretation removes the 'victim-blaming' stereotypes both of men as controlled by their lusts and animal instincts and of women as either pathetic and helpless victims or masochists who 'ask for it' by nagging (Stark *et al* 1979).

While the family is a haven of refuge for some women and men, it is a private scene of degradation for others. Stark and his colleagues ask 'Exactly what do men "win" when they beat their wives?' Images of manhood projected to them are always beyond their reach and, while blaming other individuals for their feelings of failure and ineffectualness may give passing satisfaction, violence demeans men too. Acting out hostility in this way is no more healthy than turning it inwards and becoming depressed, as women tend to do (Fransella & Frost 1977).

GENDER AND WORK

Although staying at home may be isolating, going out to work can be a mixed blessing for both women and men. Work time and pressures encroach on family life, stress-related illnesses are on the increase, and some jobs cause particular diseases, for example

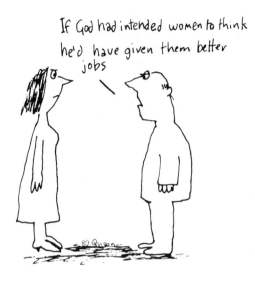

If God had intended women to think he'd have given them better jobs

pneumoconiosis in mining and byssinosis in textile industries. At the same time, going out to work has beneficial effects on health, adding to workers' self-esteem, giving a sense of meaning to their lives, and providing company and social support (Gore 1978). Women are dissatisfied with a full-time housewife role and men get depressed too when they lose their jobs or take on a house-keeping role. We have already seen that the nuclear family, with its male breadwinner and full-time housewife, is not the norm and government statistics show that over 40 per cent of the workforce are women. Most of them work for the major part of their adult lives, over half of all married women and 70 per cent of married women aged 35 to 54 going out to work (Department of Employment 1979). Their principal reason for taking a job is financial, with wanting social contacts coming second in the list of reasons (Dunnell 1979).

Women and men are concentrated in different industries in a pattern which closely mirrors culturally-valued gender roles in the home and family, so that over 90 per cent of typists, maids, nurses and sewing machinists are women, while over 90 per cent of managers, professional engineers and building workers are men. Physical strength is obviously not a relevant ground for this division of labour in managerial work, and even in manual trades machinery now exists which would allow any person to do 'heavy work', for example in the printing trade. Earnings vary too between women and men, and in 1980 women earned on average only 72 per cent as much as men, but even these figures understate the imbalance because they exclude part-time workers, who are mainly women. In fact, 40 per cent of women work part-time compared with less than 1 per cent of men, and this also excludes them from other benefits such as pensions, sick pay and holiday pay. Average hourly rates for part-time workers are 60 per cent of full-time men's rates, and 80 per cent of full-time women's rates (CIS 1981).

The origins of this division of labour between the sexes go back to well before the industrial revolution, when patriarchal, or male-dominated, families lived and worked as economic units based on the home. Male household heads had their distinct jobs and women and children had theirs and, when the industrial revolution began to separate home and work, this sexual division of labour was carried over into factories and offices. Earlier craft guilds had excluded women from learning skills and becoming guild members, and industrial trades unions continued the same process. Because women workers threatened the leading position of men in the labour force, men exerted their control in the new workplaces just as they had done in the home. Women were prevented from learning certain skills and became a reservoir of unskilled labour, as they often remain today, with very few apprenticeships and on-the-job training opportunities open to them (Beechey 1983).

Defining skilled work is problematic, however. In the last century all clerical workers were men and this was a high status, skilled and much sought-after job. As typewriters were introduced and the work became more routine these posts were increasingly given to women, so that today women are the majority of clerical workers. Deskilling of a job, when it becomes routinised and lowered in status, usually leads to its feminisation. Parallel examples may be seen in the cases of the stethoscope, sphygmomano-meter and ECG monitor. When these instruments were first invented and were technically advanced for their time their use was confined to doctors, who were mainly men. But as they became widespread they were turned over to mainly women nurses and technicians for routine use. What is a skilled job is therefore less to do with the nature of the task than a matter of social definition.

As we saw in the case of housework, jobs that are monotonous, fragmented and inflexible are unpopular and stressful for whoever does them. In the home and in paid employment women are concentrated in this kind of work, but it is a feature of working life for thousands of men too. The compensations of work are the sense of self-worth it brings, together with opportunities for stimulation and sharing one's experiences with other workers. These are some of the reasons why paying wages for housework would not be a satisfactory answer to the sexual division of labour between women and men, and between home and outside work. An insurance company has calculated that a housewife's weekly wage should be £204, or £10,600 per year, taking into account the kinds of work done and the hours involved (Barrett & McIntosh 1982), but to pay wages for housework would continue to confine people to this narrow and dissatisfying role, whether they were women or men. Wages would probably not attract large numbers of men to housework because of its nature and low status, and so paying those who did it would add legitimacy to the idea that this is women's work. Sharing tasks more equally, developing more machines to do the work, and providing more social services such as nurseries, laundries and restaurants are ways of relieving everybody of tedious and non-rewarding work which have been adopted in times of war but which could offer benefits in peace-time too.

IMAGES OF SEXUALITY

Besides the family and school, information about sexuality is presented to children at their learning stages and reinforced for adults in the way women and men are represented in books and in the media.

Analyses of children's books have shown that the sexes are not equally portrayed in quantity or quality. One study of prizewinning books found that human males were shown in pictures 11 times more often than females, but when it came to pictures of animals there were 95 males to every female (Weitzman *et al* 1976). Story lines show women and men differently too. Adventures are more likely to feature males, as in *Tarzan* and *Treasure Island*, with females placed in service roles like Snow White looking after the seven dwarfs, or in fantasy roles such as fairy godmothers or princesses. Boys are shown as more aggressive, in sporting activities and solving problems, and adult men continue to solve problems and to be in business and outdoor settings but are less aggressive. Women appear in homes and schools more often (Fransella & Frost 1977), and it is interesting that the controversy about the effects of television programmes portraying male violence is not matched by discussions of the way women are shown. Children spend more time watching television than going to school, and these representations of sexuality therefore reach extensive audiences.

Advertisements in magazines and on television and billboards feature stereotypes of femininity and masculinity along similar lines. Cigarette advertisements associate cowboys, sports and outdoor pursuits with maleness and convey images of masculinity as rugged, tough and violent. Women in advertisements are often in various stages of undress, or in dependent or domestic settings which transmit notions of them as physically provocative objects for male pleasure, or identify them predominantly as wives and mothers rather than as individuals in their own right (Fransella & Frost 1977). Women are more often shown indoors and, in a mixed group of women, men and children, women are more likely to be standing up and attending to others while men and children are seated awaiting services. Recently a new trend has appeared in advertisements, appealing to the 'liberated' woman (Beechey 1982). Women are shown more often in previously 'male' locations such as offices and in outdoor sports activities, and their sexuality is portrayed in a more active style. After meeting a man and smelling his aftershave, the liberated advertisement woman is ready for sexual passion, but essentially the image of male sexual initiative remains and the basic message has not changed.

Linking these images with our discussion of rape and wife-beating on the one hand and family and work life on the other reveals a pattern in the ways female and male sexuality is learned and lived. Women come to see themselves as dependent, emotional and providers of all kinds of services, including the sexual kind. Men learn that they are supposed to be active, independent, ambitious and high achievers in the realms of work, finances and sex. These are the ways in which gender stereotypes actually get inside people's heads, and their effects on health can be far-reaching.

SEXUALITY AND HEALTH

Are men more healthy than women or do women suffer from less illness, as their greater life expectancy might suggest? Having got thus far in our discussion we might expect things to be more complex than this, and in fact illness statistics vary not only according to sex but also with marital status, social class, employment status, race and many other factors, and the physical/mental illness split introduces even more complications.

Males have higher infant mortality rates and throughout life have more accidents and occupationally-related illness (Office of Health Economics 1978; 1979). As well as these, other diagnoses which occur more often in males also seem to be linked with different life-styles and their associated stress levels. Men have more coronary heart disease, kidney conditions and peptic ulcers. They also have higher overall rates for cancer, but whether these are related to carcinogenic chemicals or radiation, or linked with stress and other life-style factors, are still matters for speculation (Oakley 1981). Male admission rates to psychiatric hospitals are higher in categories such as alcohol and drug-induced conditions and personality disorders and, although women make more suicide attempts, men are more successful in committing suicide. From the age of 35 upwards, single men have more mental illness than single women, and employed men's rates are lower than the unemployed. Psychiatric symptoms decrease with higher education levels in men, but increase for women.

Females have higher rates of admission to psychiatric hospitals for depressive conditions but the rates for unemployed men overtake these (DHSS 1977). Working class women are five times more likely to have psychiatric illnesses than middle class women, and having small children at home, being unemployed and not having a close supporting relationship with either a woman or man increases their likelihood of psychiatric illness (Brown *et al* 1975). Single women are more mentally healthy than single men (Gove & Tudor 1972). Turning to women's physical health, their previously lower rates of coronary heart disease, peptic ulcer and conditions related to smoking and alcohol are catching up with male rates as life-styles change and more women enter certain kinds of jobs (Oliver 1974).

Common findings between women and men are that having a job is protective against mental illness, and this may be because working outside the home provides sources of social support and self-esteem which unemployed men and isolated women do not have. However, stress-related disorders increase in some kinds of work for both women and men. One suggested interpretation of women's and men's different mental illness rates is linked with cultural norms of femininity and masculinity (Chesler 1972). Females learn that it is unfeminine to express aggression and they turn their hostility and dissatisfactions inwards and become depressed, while males are encouraged to show aggression and 'strong' behaviour, which leads them to turn their hostility outwards to violence either against themselves in suicide or other forms of self-abuse like alcohol and drugs, or against others. Higher male rates of conviction for violent crimes could be interpreted in the same way.

Patients are only one side of the medical encounter, however, and a study of doctors and the way they categorise and diagnose patients has shed further light on the question of different illnesses and illness rates among women and men. Diagnosis and treatment is a process of interaction between patient and doctor, and several studies have consistently found that doctors' standards of mental health are different for women and men. Doctors tend to visualize healthy men as similar to the male sex-role stereotype of self-reliance, efficiency and rationality. Mentally healthy women are also defined in parallel with the stereotypes as emotional, sensitive, submissive and conceited but, as many critics have pointed out, this is a strange description of health (Williams 1977). When psychiatrists are asked to define a healthy adult of unspecified sex, they revert to the same characteristics they use for healthy men, which again suggests that they see masculinity as health and femininity as sickness (Broverman *et al* 1970). Whilst it is not surprising that psychiatrists share the same stereotypes as others in their culture, their notions of health and illness will colour their decisions on who is sick, what treatment to give, and how to assess recovery and return to 'health'. Our discussion of wife-battering showed that a psychiatric label is sometimes given to women's conditions when another kind of description is more appropriate, for it is not necessarily the woman herself who is 'sick'.

Further evidence that doctors as well as others see women as emotional and irrational is provided by a report about 'alleged psychogenic disorders in women' (Lennane & Lennane 1982). Doctors' explanations in medical textbooks of dysmenorrhoea, nausea of pregnancy, pain in labour and behaviour disturbances in babies located their causes in psychological problems of women, or at least said that emotional factors aggravated the conditions. These explanations were given despite the existence of well-founded evidence that the conditions had organic causes. What these doctors thought was all in the mind of the patient was more likely to be in the eye of the medical beholder, and we have also seen the part doctors' concepts of gender have played in the definition of the 'maternal instinct' and menopause-related symptoms.

Social role differences have been the focus of attempts to decide whether women and men have different illness rates and what might cause any differences, and three main variations on the theme have emerged (Nathanson 1975). The first theory suggests that women report more illness than men because cultural norms of femininity make it more acceptable for women to be ill, and this version distinguishes between 'actual' illness and whether people report to a doctor, for not all illness results in 'illness behaviour' or help-seeking from doctors. The second theory suggests that being ill, that is reporting sick and adopting a 'sick role', is more compatible with women's other role responsibilities. Evidence on this is conflicting, because women with pre-school children have low levels of reporting sick. They have the opportunity to adopt a sick role because they do not have the obligation to attend regularly at a place of employment, but their home role gives them little time to be ill because they cannot put off doing jobs like changing nappies and feeding the family. This explanation also conflicts with the third theory, which is that the greater role stress and conflict in women's roles leads to more illness. In this version, women with many responsibilities such as young children and an outside job should report more illness, not less.

Once again there is a major problem with the research methods. Researchers have confused illness and illness behaviour, and different criteria of illness have been used including hospitalisation rates, days off sick from work, number of visits to the doctor and so on. These measures are clearly not looking at the same thing, and an added complication is the way doctors make diagnoses, as we have already discussed. The only firm conclusions that can be drawn are, firstly, that differences in types and rates of illness may occur between women and men, but there are also large variations related to social class, age, marital status and family composition. Secondly, much depends not only on how people feel and the actions they take, but also on the responses of workers in the health care system.

CONCLUSION

Biological, psychological and sociological theories of sexuality, their research methods, findings and implications have been our concern so far, but the question which now has to be answered is

'Where does all this evidence leave us?' Biological differences between the sexes are obvious but the argument that they determine different ways of behaving and justify particular social arrangements is not proven. Social influences on how we live out our biology and develop our personalities are very strong, to say the least. Leaving biological differences out of the debate entirely would amount to a social reductionism, or reducing everything to social causes, and this would not stand up to the evidence any better than explaining everything in terms of biology. Even if we were to accept the 'human nature being what it is...' argument, that would not mean that present social arrangements are inevitable and unchangeable. After all, smallpox, cholera and the plague are natural phenomena but humans have still tried to find ways of ending their harmful effects on health.

Our present state of social development makes biological differences increasingly irrelevant. Heavy work can be mechanised so that everyone can do it, whether they are large or small, women or men, and improved contraception has at least freed women from repeated pregnancies if they wish this, even if a totally reliable and safe method has not yet been developed.

Social differences between women and men are no longer based on biological needs, if they ever were. These differences – which in reality are inequalities with harmful effects for all of us – are now passed on via ideas or ways of thinking about the world which we have called biological determinism. If we would like a more healthy society, then it is these ideologies or misrepresentations which we must change. As we saw at the beginning of this chapter, we are actively involved in making sense of our social world and are not just passively socialised into playing roles. Therefore we can work on changing these ideologies which disguise the way things are and which are used to persuade us to accept existing arrangements as natural and inevitable.

There is so much human diversity that to place people in one of two categories, or even at points on a line between two polar opposites of femininity and masculinity, is too limiting. People of whatever biological sex should be free to behave and live as they want with regard to gender roles and sexual preferences. The only limit that needs to exist is that their freedom, equality and self-expression does not oppress, exploit or harm others in the way that present social arrangements do in different ways for both women and men. We would then live in a much more healthy society and be more healthy as individuals too.

SECTION 2

Illness,
Disability
&
Sexuality

CHAPTER 5

Sexuality and Self-concept: Effects of Illness and Disability

People are sexual beings all the time, whether they are healthy, ill or disabled, and they experience and express their sexuality in unique, individual ways. Our review of biological, psychological and sociological perspectives on sexuality has shown that there are more similarities than differences between the sexes, and that large areas of overlap exist in women's and men's physical make-up, personalities and social lives. This means that categorising people as either female or male is useful only in limited circumstances and it is almost always more appropriate to think of them having a mixture of some of the characteristics usually defined as feminine and masculine, as well as having other attributes which are not specific to one particular sex.

Assessing ourselves and others according to stereotypes is not only inaccurate and unscientific, but can impair judgements about how to relate to others and lead to false expectations of their responses. As nurses we try to give individualised care, but we shall not succeed in this if we base our care planning on stereotypes and do things 'because we've always done it like that'. In the past we have done many things which we now know are useless or positively harmful, such as massaging pressure areas with spirit and powder. But when research demonstrated that these practices were inappropriate we struggled to abandon outdated ideas and to adopt more rational and logical ways. As professionals, we examine and criticise our actions and bring new ideas to our work so that we really do give individualised and not stereotyped patient care, and sexuality is one important area in which a great deal of re-thinking is needed.

In this chapter we shall consider how people's sexuality may be affected by *any* illness or disability, and by having treatment in hospital or at home, and later chapters will show that specific illnesses, disabilities and treatments have their own particular effects of which nurses need to be aware when planning, giving and evaluating nursing care.

SEXUALITY IN EVERYDAY LIFE

Healthy people take for granted and perhaps give little thought to aspects of daily life which are linked to sexuality. For most people, core gender identity – or a self-concept of femininity or masculinity – is settled in childhood. Although experiments with clothes and behaviour, including sexual behaviour, continue through adolescence and into adult life, fundamental changes are not made. Different aspects of gender may be emphasised at different periods, with physical appearance perhaps featuring heavily for teenagers, while parenthood and working life contribute more to adults' views of themselves as sexual beings.

Gender roles at home and at work both express and contribute to self-concept, including gender identity. Certain key roles may be the focus of people's self-definitions, and being a parent is an example of this. We have seen that parenthood has greatly varying significance in people's lives, and parental roles and the organisation of family life are carried out in a multitude of ways. Working life outside the home also plays a part in building the self-concept and is one of many factors which can build up or undermine self-esteem and feelings of personal worth. Like other aspects of life related to sexuality, the importance of social roles may only become apparent when they are lost or threatened, and infertility or unemployment can have devastating and destructive effects on both women's and men's lives.

Intimate sexual behaviour too becomes an established part of life, taking such a myriad of forms that anything and everything can be considered 'normal'. Having sex, or not having sex (celibacy), a frequency of once a week or once a year, having one or more partners of the same or different sex, and a range of acts from self-pleasuring (masturbation) through mutual stimulation to sexual intercourse are all 'normal' in the sense that plenty of other people are doing them too. Whatever is acceptable and gives pleasure and satisfaction to the people involved, and does not exploit or hurt them in any way, is normal. If any kind of sexual activity is imposed on people against their will or causes them emotional or physical injury then it is wrong, and this definition applies to every kind of behaviour. Using physical force or emotional blackmail to persuade people to do something is immoral and possibly illegal in any context, sexual or non-sexual, and sexual behaviour is not different or special in that sense.

All these aspects of sexuality in everyday life are taken for granted and may not even come into people's minds in the ordinary course of events. When illness intervenes, however, people's self-concepts and value in their own eyes and those of others may suddenly be deeply challenged.

SEXUAL SELF-CONCEPT IN ILLNESS AND DISABILITY

Operations which change physical appearance are an obvious threat to self-esteem because body image is altered for the individual and for others. Women do not feel the same after a mastectomy because they do not look the same, for example, and the sexual connotations of breasts in our culture, as well as their physiological functions, mean that a woman may feel she is no longer sexually attractive and desirable to others after this operation. Other people, particularly her sexual partner(s), may convey subtle messages about their reactions to her scar and altered appearance by what they say and do as well as by what they do not say and do. Well-intentioned hints about wearing loose clothes to hide the loss or suggestions that wearing a bikini is no longer possible can cause a great deal of distress. The woman's self-confidence in maintaining the style of dress through which she expresses her personality may be undermined, and she may withdraw from physical contact and sexual activity for fear of upsetting others. Nurses are well aware of these possibilities now, and specialist nurses and others train as mastectomy counsellors to help women to adjust to the potentially shattering experience of having a life-threatening condition which can also prejudice sexuality (Simpson & Levitt 1981; Webb 1982a).

Many other conditions than the obvious one of mastectomy can be just as devastating for sexuality because they too change body image, whether the physical changes are outward and visible or internal and hidden. Amputations, stoma formation and drug treatments leading to hair loss can be very similar in their effects to mastectomy because they change physical appearance and may make the individual feel unattractive. Other conditions involving no change in external appearance can nevertheless affect body image. Someone who is incontinent may feel dirty and repulsive to others, while those recovering from a heart attack may view their body as weakened or inadequate in comparison with their former self-picture (Wilson-Barnett 1982). Having a visible birth-mark or other congenital abnormality such as prominent ears or limb deformities can make people insecure in their body image and aware that others may think of them as 'abnormal', and this may make them feel unwanted as friends and sexual partners.

Body image is related to the concept of wholeness, and any loss of part of the body can therefore affect the individual's picture of the self. If this change is defined as negative and an impairment, the person will feel less valued by themselves and by others, and will have these doubts unless and until others demonstrate that they still value the individual. They can give this social support in both expressive and instrumental ways (Stone *et al.* 1979; Norbeck 1981). Showing an interest in people, spending time listening and talking to them, joining in activities with them, touching and demonstrating affection all convey to people that they are wanted and needed, and that they are part of a social network of mutual responsibility, obligations and caring. Instrumental support by giving material aid conveys similar messages of empathy and caring, and in addition provides aid in the form of help with jobs, financial assistance, and equipment to promote independence and mobility. Welfare provisions including home helps, laundry ser-vices, money benefits and community nursing services also come into this category.

When people are unwell or disabled, they may have to rely on others to a varying extent for help in maintaining their body image. Personal hygiene, arranging the hair, and dressing all contribute to body image, and people express their personalities through their appearance. Relying on others to do these things, especially if this extends to choosing and buying clothes because one cannot do this oneself, is a gross curtailment of personal autonomy and individual choice no matter how appreciative one is of sympathetic help. But if decisions like these are based on impersonal choice of clothing by an institution like a long-stay hospital, or if attendants arrange the hair in a purely functional style or one which differs from the person's usual preference, this is a violation of individuality and sexuality.

Self-esteem is the result of a positive self-concept and body image, and for most people it is linked to ideas of independence, autonomy and decision-making. People who are obliged to adopt the sick role on either a short-term or long-term basis give up to some degree their ability to be self-directing and self-caring. Some loss of independence is inevitable in certain situations, for example during early recovery from a heart attack or serious operation, or when there is permanent disability such as quadriplegia. Autonomy and self-assertion are aspects of our culturally-defined notions of sexuality, as we saw in Section 1, and whatever kind of gender identity people have, deprivation of self-determination will tend to lower their self-esteem. Care of large numbers of people in institutions has often led to 'batch' treatment and 'processing' in a way which is convenient for the institution but which takes away individual autonomy (Goffman 1963). A particularly telling example of this is reported by Francis Cohen, who studied recovery from surgery and compared patients who sought information and tried to control their progress with other patients who were relatively passive in hospital (Cohen & Lazarus 1973). Those who tried to be more autonomous, for example by asking for pain-relieving drugs, had more 'negative psychological reactions' and a generally more complicated post-operative course. It seems that hospital staff viewed patients' attempts to control their own situations as abnormal and Cohen concluded that adopting a passive role in hospital may be a more rational strategy because staff expect this and cope better when patients meet their expectations.

Individualised patient care is now being more widely practised and this should mean that individuals exercise more influence over their own care and take part in decisions about what is or is not done to and for them. Assisting and encouraging people to decide for themselves what their treatment should be, and then to be self-caring within the constraints of their illness or disability, acknowledges and respects their sexuality as part of their individuality, and contributes towards a positive self-concept.

SEXUALITY AND PRIVACY

Expressing emotion is linked with sexuality and different cultures have their own norms and values about appropriate ways of releasing tension and of demonstrating affection, anger, frustration and other moods. Within our culture, stereotypes of femininity and masculinity define emotional release as acceptable or even expected for women, while men are encouraged to be more emotionally self-contained, as we saw in Section 1. A more personalised approach, however, would be concerned with assessing people's different emotional needs and responses and assist-ing them to cope in the most constructive way for them as individuals.

Illness or disability may bring great emotional pressures and consequently people need to be able to think about their situation, sometimes in total privacy and sometimes with those close to them or with professionals, but whether patients or clients are cared for at home or in hospital, their privacy is likely to be greatly restricted. In hospital most patients share a room with others by day and night, and the space between beds may not be great enough to allow confidential discussions. If visitors are enter-tained in the day room the same problem occurs, and private rooms are almost never available for visiting. Facilities in hospital can make any show of emotion embarrassing because of the public nature of the setting. It can be very difficult for patients to have a good laugh with their visitors for fear of upsetting or disturbing others, but how much more necessary it is sometimes to have a good cry, a hug or a heated debate to help take difficult decisions. Failing to look for ways to make these possible in a relaxed atmosphere is another side of institutional failure to respect sexuality and individuality.

Professionals are frequently obliged to take personal histories in a setting where overhearing is likely and patients' emotional priva-cy is thereby invaded. When out-patients wait in various stages of undress in view of other patients and staff not directly involved with them, or curtains round beds are not pulled quite far enough to prevent overlooking by passers-by, both physical and emotion-al privacy are compromised. Procedures involving exposure of parts of the body which are usually covered amount to an invasion of personal space which is even more intrusive when body orifices are entered during physical examinations or when conducting technical procedures. The whole body belongs to the individual, and modesty and sexuality are threatened when *any* part is exposed, because emotions and sexual feelings do not pertain only to genital organs.

Physical expressions of sexuality take forms from simple eye contact, smiles, kissing on the cheek and holding hands right through to genital sex acts, and sick or disabled people's sexual needs are the same as those of everyone else. In acute sickness other needs and concerns temporarily assume over-riding import-ance but, as soon as recovery begins, patients often have increased needs for reassurance that they can still feel and give sexual pleasure, and mastectomy and heart attack are two examples where this may happen. Communicating these feelings verbally and non-verbally is highly problematic in hospitals and residential institutions because people are sensitive to others' reactions and afraid of embarrassment. Imagining the likely result if patients were to pull the curtains to shield their bed spaces during visiting time confirms that their fears of embarrassment are well-founded! Even when patients are nursed in single rooms their privacy may be only marginally increased, because it is not customary to knock on the door and wait for a reply before entering. Often the door of a single room is kept open or an unscreened window in the door inhibits privacy.

Sick or disabled people living at home may be no better off than those in institutions with regard to personal space and freedom to express themselves emotionally and physically. They may sleep in the family living room in order to be downstairs with others, but they thereby give up all privacy in exchange for the pleasure of company. Overcrowding may prevent a client having an individual room at home, and an opportunity to entertain visitors alone may be rare or impossible to arrange. A common myth is that older people or handicapped people lose their sexuality and are somehow asexual (Weinberg 1982) but the reality is more likely to be that their circumstances permit them little or no chance to express their sexuality in all its aspects.

EMOTIONAL REACTIONS AND SEXUALITY

Emotions and sexuality affect each other in a reciprocal or two-way manner. Negative moods such as depression and irritability are likely to dampen other emotional responses including sexual responses and, by the same token, lack of opportunity for sexual expression may have adverse emotional consequences.

Emotional debility is an aspect of virtually all illness and disability, but its extent will vary according to the meaning of the condition for the patient or client as well as depending on the severity of the condition (Lazarus 1966). Depression after a bout of influenza, or resentment and frustration at having a broken arm in plaster, will soon pass but may have a transitory effect on sexuality, perhaps by making the sufferer feel unattractive, dependent on others for assistance with body functions, or unable to carry out usual roles. More severe or long-lasting illness or permanent handicap can have profound implications for sexuality because people then have to adjust to a new self-concept and new social status, which can mean finding new ways of expressing sexuality in all its forms, including sexual acts. This re-learning process can be long, drawn out and fraught with set-backs and frustrations, so that phases of severe depression are not uncommon (Wilson-Barnett 1982).

Unpleasant mood states form a complex made up of depression, anxiety, tension, guilt, resentment and hostility (Beck 1968) and any or all of these can be attributed to threats to or disturbances of sexuality both in health and illness or disability. For example, road accident victims with facial scars, broken limbs and fractured pelvices will be anxious that their recovery may be incomplete or take a long time. The prospect of an extended stay in hospital, with its loss of independence and privacy, may lead to irritability and depression. There may be elements of resentment and hostility about why the accident happened to them or perhaps they may feel guilty if it was partly their fault. They will feel unattractive to others while bruising and stitches are still present, but fear of permanent scarring may add to the depressing feeling of perhaps not being sexually desirable to others or being so disabled that sexual activity will never be possible again.

The specific sexual aspects of some illnesses or disabilities are particularly likely to lead to feelings of guilt and depression if people blame their own past sexual behaviour for their condition. Cancer and other diseases of the genital tract may cause people to wonder if they have contributed to their own problems, for example by having a number of sexual partners or by carrying out sexual practices of which others might disapprove, such as masturbation or oral sex. Religious teaching and beliefs may be involved in guilt reactions, particularly where strict prohibitions exist on pre- or extra-marital sexual relations, and people may interpret their illness as a punishment for past 'sins' (Hogan 1980; Weinberg 1982).

Emotional and behavioural reactions with a more openly sexual aspect can occur because patients or clients feel that their sexuality is threatened. Sexual joking or unwanted touching and other sexual advances may originate from denial that sexuality is threatened, or from attempts to over-compensate for feelings of inadequacy by 'acting out' sexually. Patients may be trying to provoke a response from staff to sexual advances in order to prove to themselves that other people still find them attractive or to demonstrate that they continue to have sexual feelings and needs. Sexual or 'dirty' jokes may be the only link with sexuality which is possible in an institutional setting which offers no opportunities for freedom of expression and behaviour, particularly where people are confined for long periods. Staff may find this irritating, but when interpreted as an attempt by patients to bring sexuality into the open, perhaps in an effort to gain information, it indicates an unmet need which nurses could fill. Joining in with joking or ignoring it are ways of coping for both staff and patients, but they do not deal with the underlying questions, and ignoring sexuality is one form of information-giving. It implies that, as nothing has been said, there is nothing to say and no problems to confront.

SEXUALITY: NEEDS OF PATIENTS AND CLIENTS

Knowledge and non-judgemental attitudes are what patients and clients need from nurses, and the two go together. When staff are knowledgeable about sexuality and secure in their own sexuality, they are more comfortable in dealing with the sexual aspects of their work (Payne 1976). Knowledge of the biological, psychological and social bases of behaviour reveals the wide range of 'normality' and forms of self-identity and behaviour which exist within different cultures and in our own society. Everyone has personal values and standards regarding sexuality as well as other areas of life, and nurses are not required to give up or change their beliefs in order to carry out their professional role. But extending the same freedoms to others depends on knowledge about their beliefs and behaviour, and acknowledgement of them in a non-judgemental way.

Young women need counselling and information about contraception before and after abortion, for example, and heterosexual and homosexual patients of all ages need advice about sexuality after operations like hysterectomy or prostatectomy. Women with young children and paid employment need to discuss how to combine their two roles when they are recovering from illness or learning to live with disability. These are just a few examples of instances where nurses' personal values may be at variance with those of their patients, but where the ethic of professional neutrality should operate (United Kingdom Central Council 1983). Recognising, acknowledging and accepting one's own judgemental feelings, not suppressing or changing them, is the way to develop security and openness in dealing with controversial questions like these (Goldsborough 1970).

Awareness of the complexities of sexuality is an essential basis for assessing patients' and clients' needs for nursing care, planning and carrying out nursing interventions, and evaluating their effects. Sexuality and its possible implications and repercussions in all illnesses and disabilities have been the focus of this chapter, and the discussion has included self-concept, body image, self-esteem, and how these may be built up by positive social support or damaged by loss of independence, control and privacy. In the next chapters we shall go on to examine how sexuality is affected by particular diseases, disabilities and treatments and to see the great potential for developing the role of the nurse in relation to sexuality in health care.

CHAPTER 6

Sexuality in Illness and Disability

Illness and disability influence sexuality via their effects on self-concept, body image, self-esteem and social roles. A changed view of the self, reflected and reinforced by other people's reactions, can cause emotional disturbances ranging from feeling 'low' to overt clinical depression accompanied by a variety of other unpleasant mood states including anxiety and hostility. Mood and physical states have a feedback relationship with each other, with depression leading to physiological changes and vice versa. Depression involves lowered energy levels, insomnia, appetite disturbance, loss of libido or sexual energy, and possibly impotence or loss of capacity to have orgasms, while physiological disturbances reflect back on emotional states and can make unpleasant moods worse (Beck 1968). A vicious spiral may be set in motion, with physical and emotional debility augmenting each other at every turn. The sufferer feels unwell, tired and disinterested in the self and others, anticipates that others can see this and may withdraw their support and affection, and this causes a further fall in self-esteem. Anyone who has experienced an episode of depression after a bout of influenza or glandular fever will appreciate how illness can have these results on energy levels, including sexual energy.

As well as these basic biopsychosocial problems of disturbed self-concept, body image and the loss of independence and privacy which we discussed in Chapter 5, additional special problems will occur for patients or clients depending on which body system is disturbed or malfunctioning. In this chapter, particular aspects of sexuality related to illness and disability will

75

be analysed on the basis of the body system principally concerned, but we shall keep returning to the fact that people are biopsychosocial beings, and that the physical, emotional and sexual effects of illness and disability are therefore interwoven. This makes it difficult to divide problems neatly into categories. Should diarrhoea be considered as a disturbance of the digestive system, for example, or does it make more sense to group it with urinary problems as a disturbance of elimination because it can share many common features for patients, such as embarrassment or feeling dirty? Any classification system is therefore arbitrary, but for nurses the main concern is with problems as they affect patients or clients. Therefore our discussion will focus on patient or client problems related to sexuality, arranged according to the body system principally involved in the physiological malfunction under consideration.

SEXUALITY AND THE SKIN

Our skin is one of the most visible features we have, and its role in our lives goes far beyond the protective functions which we normally take for granted. Finding a new spot on the face when washing in the morning is enough to ruin the whole day, and body image and mood are immediately disrupted. The person thinks that the tiny blemish is much larger and obvious to others than it really is, and feels ugly and unpleasant to be with. Other people may not even notice the spot, however. Advertisers play on and build up insecurities about 'wholeness' and portray images of an attractive appearance as fresh, unmarked and well-proportioned for both women and men. We are so heavily confronted by these expectations that they become incorporated into our perceptual framework and we therefore come to view any blemishes or irregularities in ourselves and others as defects.

Teenage acne is well-known and commercially exploited because of the disturbing effects it has on self-concept and relationships by making sufferers feel ugly, unclean and sexually repulsive. Any person having a skin disorder, scar or birthmark may experience similar emotions but these may be more devastating when the lesion is longer-lasting or permanent. Cultural expectations of beauty and handsomeness drive many people to invest a great deal of money, time, emotional and physical suffering in trying to 'improve' their appearance with creams and lotions, electrolysis, laser therapy and surgery. These attempts to attain a picture of oneself that conforms to cultural prescriptions of wholeness contrasts ironically with efforts in other cultures to achieve precisely the same objective by causing scars and marks by cutting the skin of the face and other parts of the body, or using lip-plates to stretch the lips. In any setting difference becomes deviance, and much suffering is caused to those who do not match up to expected standards. People view themselves and others as objects to be admired or otherwise rather than human beings who are worthwhile whatever their superficial appearance may be.

Hair, as an appendage of the skin, is closely involved in similar notions of suitability and beauty. The 'right' amount of body hair differs for women and men, with women bleaching, shaving or otherwise removing hair from the very places on their faces and breasts where men are cultivating it as a sign of sexuality. When people lose their hair completely or it becomes thinner with ageing, different standards apply for women and men too. Balding in men is jokingly referred to as a sign of increased virility but a woman with thinning hair is to be pitied. Loss of hair as a result of illness, drugs or radiation treatment can be devastating to the individual, whose appearance not only diminishes her sense of attractiveness but is an ever-present reminder of her illness.

People who have chronic or permanent skin disorders, then, are likely to feel dissatisfied with their appearance and unattractive or even repellent to others as companions or sexual partners. Many people think that all skin diseases are contagious and therefore try to avoid close contact with sufferers for fear of 'catching' the disease themselves. This is rarely possble, and dermatologists are taught to touch and handle their patients' skins to reassure them that they are not infectious or unpleasant to be close to. If a skin condition causes itching, burning or other unpleasant sensations this will add to the negative emotions already caused by feeling ugly and may induce the sufferer to withdraw even more from social contacts. Insecurity and isolation will then further add to depression and feelings of unworthiness, and the vicious circle goes round another turn.

This complex of emotions in sufferers from skin conditions and people they encounter in daily life may have deep effects on self-concept and body image and make it hard for people to conform to norms of sexual attractiveness and meet possible sexual partners. Feelings of unattractiveness and depression are provoked which may diminish desire for sexual activity, and fears of passing on disorders to children may mar sexual enjoyment.

People may feel driven to withdraw from social life and may engage in elaborate attempts to disguise or hide their 'defects', at great cost to themselves in emotional energy, time and money.

SEXUALITY AND THE NEUROMUSCULAR SYSTEM

The principal problems faced by people with disorders of the neuromuscular system are complete or partial immobility, loss of strength and function, pain and deformity. Arthritis is perhaps the commonest cause of dysfunction in this system, osteoarthritis affecting virtually everyone to some degree as the ageing process advances. The chronic pain of arthritis is debilitating both physically and emotionally, leading to fatigue, general malaise and a variety of adverse mood states including anger and hostility, but most notably depression. Recurrent pain focuses a great deal of mental energy on to its management and can cause its sufferer to become self-centred, withdrawn or demanding. Relationships with others will inevitably be disrupted, particularly where the sufferer has to rely on relatives and friends for personal care. Decreased mobility and strength may call for alterations in role functions at home and at work, and loss of independence, earning power and social status will erode self-esteem.

Arthritis sufferers who are in frequent pain, limited in their movements and have joint deformities may perceive themselves as less able to take part in sexual activities both because of physical limitations and because they suspect their condition prevents others from finding them attractive. This complex of physical and psychosocial influences may easily depress libido further, and the side-effects of steroid drugs can add to feelings of unattractiveness. Hip joints, knees, shoulders, elbows and hands are all involved in genital sex acts as well as non-genital sexual activity including touching and hugging, and an arthritis sufferer may also be restricted in self-pleasuring by masturbation.

Many other conditions affecting the neuromuscular system cause similar or related problems for sexuality, and muscular dystrophies, amputations, strokes and spinal cord injuries are some of these.

Cerebrovascular accidents can cause physical and psychosocial problems related to sexuality. Varying degrees of paralysis affect body image and self-esteem, as well as interfering with activities of all kinds from work, household and social activities to sexual acts. The brain area responsible for libido may be affected by the cerebral infarction and memory, speech and disturbances in perception may also occur. Body image and self-concept are likely to be profoundly negatively affected, and post-stroke depression may persist for some time. This, together with loss of independence and autonomy in self-care and mobility, can lead to frustration and feelings of humiliation which will further undermine self-esteem. Nursing care aimed at regaining maximal independence and preserving dignity therefore contributes to promoting a return to pre-stroke levels in sexuality as in all other aspects of daily living, and involvement and continued support by family and friends will help the sufferer to feel worthwhile and desired as a person and sexual being. Speech therapy plays a role here, too, because ability to communicate with others is vital for maintaining social and sexual relationships.

Paralysed people have to learn to adapt the way they carry out sexual activities just as they need to do with walking, eating and dressing, and this is above all a question of experimenting with a sympathetic partner in a relaxed atmosphere and trying to maintain a sense of humour in overcoming potential frustrations and embarrassments. It may be that experiments with non-genital sexual activity and mutual self-pleasuring rather than genital sex acts will be a solution for some post-stroke people.

Problems experienced by spinal cord-injured (SCI) patients or clients mirror those of the neuromuscular disorders already discussed, with an additional exacerbating factor being that the majority of these people will be relatively young. Most spinal cord injuries are caused by trauma such as a car or work accident or fall during sporting or leisure activities. The devastating effect on the total self-concept, including its sexual side, are then all the greater because of the lost potential in family, work, social and sexual life.

Depression is a common response which may last for varying periods and be increased or replaced by anger, resentment, guilt or self-blame as well as hostility towards helpers, both informal and professional, on whom the person has to rely for intimate bodily functions and services. Mobility and independence are compromised, bowel and bladder control may be partially or totally lost, and skin breakdown is a risk and may cause painful and infected sores. Many everyday activities have to be managed in a new way and adjustment may taken many months or years.

To say that self-concept and sexuality will be undermined by such a shattering experience is a platitude. Social relationships may have to be rebuilt from a new basis and long-lasting friendships, especially sexual ones, may not survive the upheaval. Work and leisure activities will be impeded for some time and major new roles may have to be learned. Work with the former degree of responsibility, status and pay may no longer be possible, making financial self-support as difficult to achieve as independent personal care. This complex of inter-related physical and emotional threats will undoubtedly severely affect sexual desire and feelings of attractiveness, but in addition sexual function will be impaired to a degree which depends on the site of the SCI.

Injuries to the cervical cord cause paralysis in all four limbs (quadriplegia), while thoracic and lumbar injuries lead to paralysis of the lower limbs (paraplegia). The extent of disability depends both on the level and degree of SCI. In men, if the cord is completely interrupted both erection and ejaculation may be lost but if some fibres remain intact there is a chance of retaining sexual function. However, psychological stimuli are necessary for sexual activity and these may be temporarily or permanently lost if the self-concept is severely damaged by the SCI. On the other hand, some men with complete cord lesions have psychogenic erections, with stimuli from the brain bypassing the injured section of the cord by means of autonomic fibres. Reflex erections may occur if the lumbar and sacral parts of the cord are still complete, but these spasms may be too short and unpredictable to permit intercourse. Complete interruption of the lumbar or sacral segments causes loss of fertility for, even if ejaculation occurs, sperm are fewer and immobile and retrograde ejaculation (into the bladder) may occur.

Complete cord lesions in women lead to absence of the sensations of orgasm, but many women achieve psychogenic orgasm by using erotic fantasies. SCI women usually have an initial phase of amenorrhoea for some months and when periods return their regularity may be different. Fertility remains intact and therefore contraception is a question which sexually active SCI women need to consider. A vaginal delivery is usually possible, and contractions will be normal but labour painless if the lesion is above the level of the tenth thoracic vertebra. All women with SCI can breast-feed normally.

Both women and men with SCI may have to contend with a number of additional impediments to sexual activity, in the form of urinary catheters and collecting bags, stomas, pressure sores, deformities resulting from contractures, and painful muscular spasms. Specialist counselling can help them to adapt to their altered self-concept, body image and sexuality, and a range of specific treatments to facilitate sexual activity are available. New techniques for arousal and foreplay may need to be learned by couples, either from sex therapists or by personal experimentation. Erotic stimulation can come from music, pictures, conversations, touching and stroking those erogenous zones which retain sensation or have heightened sensations after the injury. Electric vibrators can help to bring about a response, and experiment will be needed to find the most sensitive areas. Sex therapists will be able to teach techniques for producing reflex erections and maintaining penile tumescence. Ways of managing urinary and stoma appliances will be discussed later in this chapter in the section on eliminatory systems.

Throughout our discussions, emphasis has been placed on total sexuality and the fact that what is normal, acceptable and pleasurable is a question of social and personal definition rather than immutable 'facts'. It is particularly important to remember that, for SCI people as for all of us, sexual pleasure and fulfilment comes from doing what pleases us and our partners and does not cause them pain, embarrassment and distress. What outsiders may define as 'normal' is therefore irrelevant to a couple in an intimate relationship. In a secure emotional environment SCI people with long-term problems requiring sexual adaptations can feel free to experiment with a variety of techniques, positions and sources of pleasure, both genital and non-genital, for themselves and their partners.

SEXUALITY AND THE RESPIRATORY SYSTEM

Breathlessness is the cardinal symptom of disturbed respiratory function, and difficulty in breathing may occur even at rest when disease is severe or advanced. Patients may be able to breathe satisfactorily only in a sitting position (orthopnoea) and anxiety about not being able to breathe will be increased if this position cannot be maintained. Decreased oxygen levels and correspondingly increased carbon dioxide levels in the blood cause feelings of tiredness and impair concentration, while continued coughing, which may be painful, adds to exhaustion. Along with a cough, production of sputum gives an unpleasant taste in the mouth, and breathing through the mouth causes a dry mouth and lips. Patients experience some or all of these problems to varying degrees if they have acute chest infections, chronic obstructive airways disease or malignant conditions of the respiratory tract, and pleural effusion can add to difficulty in breathing and be extremely painful.

This group of problems has major implications for all aspects of sexuality. Someone whose movements are severely restricted by breathlessness is less able to take an interest and be independent in keeping up personal appearance. Washing and combing the hair may be a huge effort and coughing, halitosis, sweating and cyanosis or flushed appearance can make the person feel uncomfortable about themselves and unappealing to others. Inability to undertake usual activities of daily living unaided, share household jobs or go out to work will diminish self-esteem, especially if the curtailment is permanent. Respiratory problems of this kind may affect adults in mid-life who would normally be relatively active and may have responsibility for supporting children, partners or relatives, and their feelings of inadequacy may be made worse by guilt if they have been smokers, or by hostility and resentment if theirs is an occupationally-induced disease.

Physical and emotional aspects may combine to affect sexual activity particularly severely for patients or clients suffering from breathlessness and its associated problems. A constant struggle to breathe may very effectively drive all thoughts of sex from the mind, or physical ability to take part in sexual acts may be greatly decreased or even eliminated by breathlessness and inability to adopt non-upright positions. Breathlessness is always accompanied by some degree of anxiety, and fear may be a great deterrent to sexual activity because existing dyspnoea will be increased as the respiratory rate increases in the excitement, plateau and orgasm phases of sexual acts (Masters & Johnson 1965). A sexual partner may be able to alleviate difficulties by adopting a more active role so that the breathless person is minimally exerted, and experiments with alternative positions and additional pillows for support can help. Sexual intercourse may be impossible, however, and other forms of sexual activity may replace this, for example mutual genital pleasuring without penetration, non-genital stimulation by a partner, or self-pleasuring.

Advanced respiratory disorders can lead to complete cessation of sexual activity, and this can be an extremely detrimental addition to existing self-concept damage as well as straining relationships. In this event, other aspects of sexuality assume even greater importance, and building self-esteem through maintaining appearance, dignity, independence and privacy can attempt partially to compensate for the loss of this core element of personhood.

SEXUALITY AND THE CARDIOVASCULAR SYSTEM

Myocardial infarction is probably the most common source of disturbances of sexuality related to the cardiovascular system. Heart attacks tend to occur in men at a time of life when earning a living and supporting a family are important cultural indicators of manliness. Therefore, a man who is at risk or has had a heart attack may feel that his body image is damaged and with it his self-esteem. Those with physically demanding jobs may well be advised to change to a lighter occupation but may be unable to find a suitable job, which can lead to feelings of demoralisation which further undermine self-confidence.

Problems of adjustment after a heart attack are more likely to have emotional than physical causes (Puksta 1977). Anxiety about over-exertion augments an already stressful and threatening situation, and post-infarct depression is common. Depression and anxiety can also affect the partner, usually a woman, whose own anxiety may lead her to be over-protective and reinforce her partner's fears. Anxiety and depression will dampen sexual desire and inhibit performance for both partners, which may lead to frustration and bad-temperedness for both people in a sexual partnership.

After a heart attack, the majority of patients can return to work in two or three months, and resume social and leisure activities which do not cause excessive increases in heart rate and blood pressure. In practice, the individual is the best judge of what is appropriate and a rapid heart rate and respirations, or palpitations lasting more than 15 minutes after activity, chest pain, or extreme fatigue are warning signs of too much activity. Avoiding or drastically reducing work and social contacts will probably add to depression because the consequent deprivation of social support will mean that the post-infarct patient has few opportunities to meet new people, including sexual partners if this is desired. Social isolation removes the possibility of positive reinforcement of self-image and building self-esteem by receiving feedback from other people.

Guidelines for resuming sexual activity are the same as those for other kinds of activity, and the patient should be advised to consult a doctor if palpitations and breathlessness persist 15 minutes after sexual intercourse, if chest pain occurs during or after intercourse, or extreme fatigue or difficulty in sleeping result (Weinberg 1982). Studies have shown that having sex is approximately as physically demanding as climbing 2 flights of stairs in 20 seconds (11 steps per flight, each step 6.5 inches high). People who can do this without discomfort can safely have sexual intercourse. No particular position has been found to be more or less stressful than another and masturbation is only marginally less demanding. It seems that stress surrounding sexual activity is more problematic than the sex act itself, and people should therefore avoid physical and emotional stress caused by eating a large meal, drinking a lot of alcohol, having sex when already tired or tense, and situations likely to induce 'performance anxiety' (Puksta 1977).

Drugs taken to relieve hypertension or depression can affect sexuality after a myocardial infarction and patients should be warned about this possibility (See Chapter 7), while breathlessness and dyspnoea related to cardiovascular conditions bring similar problems to those already discussed in connection with the respiratory system.

Peripheral vascular disease resulting in amputation affects all aspects of sexuality in very profound ways. The alteration in body image is very obvious to the individual and others and depression, with its attendant effects on sexual desire and feelings of self-worth, will probably be experienced to a varying extent by all amputees at first. Recurrent bouts of depression may persist if they define their loss as making them unattractive as companions and sexual partners, and they may be reluctant to try to resume sexual activities because their prosthesis or stump causes embarrassment. Amputees may feel insecure about being able to adopt and maintain for long enough positions which make sexual intercourse possible and enjoyable. They and their partners may need to experiment with positioning until they find what is comfortable, pleasurable and natural in their new situations, and until feelings of awkwardness are overcome.

Problems experienced in relation to sexuality by those with dysfunctions of the cardiovascular system have many overlaps with other body system disturbances. We have noted this in connection with respiratory problems and immobility, but other sections of this and the following chapters will also be relevant, as we shall see when we consider the unwanted side-effects of drugs used to treat cardiovascular disorders in Chapter 7.

SEXUALITY AND THE DIGESTIVE SYSTEM

The teeth are needed for the first stage of digestion but in addition they play a part in speech and make a highly visible contribution to physical appearance. People without teeth or properly-fitting dentures not only cannot digest their food efficiently and have to eat selectively, avoiding hard or tough foods, but also have changed facial appearances and speech. Absence of teeth or not wearing dentures can thus have effects on self-concept. Body image is altered, probably for the worse in the view of the self and others, and consequently self-esteem is damaged. Older people are most likely to experience these difficulties but this does not lessen their magnitude, because elderly people have sexual needs related to presentation of self and forming close relationships, as well as a continuing interest in sex acts which stereotypes often deny (Weinberg 1982). The loss of dignity they suffer if this and other aspects of their sexuality are ignored is just as damaging as it would be for a younger person.

Certain problems affecting the digestive system are related to sexuality both because they have implications for social and sexual relations and because they are more prevalent in one sex than the other. Stress-related disorders which occur differentially among women and men seem linked to occupational and other life-style factors, and to expectations of appropriate behaviour for women and men.

Pain in the upper abdomen due to 'indigestion', frank peptic ulceration or gastritis are more common in men, whose working lives may subject them to emotional pressure and strain so that they smoke more and drink more alcohol than women, as well as being unable to have regular meal-breaks. However, there is evidence that when women take up similar occupations and become subject to the same pressures and social expectations, their incidence of stress-related disorders begins to approach that of men (Oakley 1981).

Pain associated with digestive system disturbances may be accompanied by vomiting, diarrhoea or constipation, and all these problems will leave their sufferers feeling weak and unwell. This general malaise and lowered energy levels will affect all activities, including sexual activity, and the need to modify eating and drinking habits or make frequent or sudden visits to the lavatory will interfere with social activities and sexual relationships. People affected by these problems may feel unable to go out for a meal or a drink to socialise with friends for fear of getting an attack of symptoms and causing embarrassment to themselves and their companions.

Drinking alcohol can be related to sexuality both as cause and effect. Images of manliness in our culture are linked to drinking alcohol and men have higher rates of alcohol-related illness, although this problem is increasing for women too. 'Drowning your sorrows' for men may be a way of relieving work-stresses and suppressing emotions they are not able to talk about, while for women it seems to be the stress of the housewife role which leads to alcoholism (Oakley 1981). The effects of alcohol on sexuality are the reverse of what is often imagined or hoped for! Alcohol depresses the central nervous system and with it sexual capacity and pleasure. Although inhibitions may be removed and people may feel more relaxed, men experience difficulty in getting an erection and in ejaculating and women are also aroused less easily (Hogan 1980). Chronic alcoholism in men leads to gynaecomastia (increase in breast size), impotence due to peripheral nervous involvement, lowerered testosterone and increased oestrogen levels, but its effects on women have not been so extensively studied as the problem has, up to now, been diagnosed less frequently in females.

A group of problems termed 'eating disorders' occurs more often in women, but their incidence in men may be greater than was previously thought because certain diagnostic 'labels' are more readily attached to women. Anorexia nervosa, or 'The Art of Starvation' (Macleod 1981), and bulimia nervosa (self-induced vomiting alternating with eating 'binges') are diagnosed more frequently in young women who are preoccupied and dissatisfied with their physical appearance. They have distorted body images, conceiving of themselves as much heavier and fatter than they actually are. The 'ideal woman' has traditionally been self-denying and passive, giving the best food to her husband and children and denying her own needs. In parallel, female sexuality has been defined, at least in post-Freudian times, as passive and women's sexual needs as less than men's, and anorexia nervosa can be viewed as an exaggerated form of this 'normal' femininity (Oakley 1981). Thinking along the same lines, Susie Orbach in her book

'Fat is a Feminist Issue' (Orbach 1978) suggests that women who overeat and grow fat are trying to avoid being identified as 'ideal' women. Women may be portrayed in advertisements as objects of 'conspicuous consumption', their clothes and jewellery giving evidence of the wealth and success of their husbands (de Beauvoir 1960) and this too pressurises them towards stereotyped images of beauty as a thin body, with prominent bones and hollows around the neck and cheeks.

These eating disorders are 'sociosomatic' disorders because it is social expectations which induce people to embark on their self-destructive courses (Roberts 1981). They are dangerous and highly complex conditions, and specialist books should be consulted by those who wish to know more about the subject.

SEXUALITY AND THE ENDOCRINE SYSTEM

The endocrine system protects the body by helping to maintain its internal equilibrium in physical and psychological terms, hormones being involved in processes ranging from metabolism to stress reactions. A number of dysfunctions of the endocrine system can cause problems for sexuality, both in the broad sense of gender identity and roles and in the narrower sense of sexual acts.

Diabetes mellitus is probably the most common endocrine disorder affecting sexuality (Hogan 1980) because the degenerative problems of the circulatory, nervous and renal systems which may affect the health of diabetics can lead to difficulties in sexual function such as loss of libido, impotence and ejaculatory incompetence. The basic disturbance of pancreatic function, necessitating changes in diet and perhaps taking insulin or oral drugs, causes potential problems by threatening the self-concept of a whole and healthy individual, and adaptations in life-style are needed to ensure that balanced blood sugar levels are maintained through regular eating habits. As control is gained, disruptions can virtually disappear or can be managed so that social life is not interfered with, but anxiety about hypoglycaemic attacks may inhibit diabetics and their companions from perceiving them as 'normal' and sexual persons.

The effects of diabetes on the male reproductive system have been more extensively studied and are therefore better understood than its effects on women (Hogan 1980, Woods 1984). Impotence, retrograde ejaculation and infertility are all increased in incidence in male diabetics, but the cause is not clear and is likely to be a combination of vascular, neurological and psychogenic factors. Diabetics have more extensive atherosclerotic changes than non-diabetics and blockage of the small blood vessels supplying the corpus cavernosa may interfere with the blood supply required for erection, while libido and ability to have an orgasm remain. Diabetic neuropathy of the parasympathetic system leads to impotence, and sympathetic involvement interferes with ejaculation and possibly also with erection. Retrograde ejaculation may be a cause of infertility, and occurs in 1–2 per cent of diabetic men (Kolodny *et al* 1979). It results from autonomic neuropathy at the site of the bladder neck, where the internal sphincter no longer closes fully and semen can thus enter the bladder, mix with urine and be expelled during micturition.

It can be very difficult to distinguish psychogenic impotence from that caused by physiological changes. For all men, psychological factors are paramount in sexual arousal and performance, and therefore emotional influences can affect sexual activity. If erectile or ejaculatory problems develop for physiological reasons, psychological factors will come into effect too, because of fear of failure and loss of a sense of masculinity due to inability to perform sexual acts. Even with no physiological changes, a diabetic man's sense of manhood may be threatened if life-style changes are needed as a result of the condition, and this disturbance of self-concept may be enough to compromise sexual functioning.

The extent of orgasm disturbance in women diabetics is not clear, but there is evidence that they do have an increased incidence of dysfunction compared with non-diabetics. As with male problems, the causes are likely to be one or more vascular, neurological and psychosocial factors. However, diabetic women are more susceptible to vaginal infections, which result in soreness and dryness, as well as possibly having reduced vaginal lubrication due to vascular or neurological changes. Pain or difficulty during intercourse has a deterrent effect on sexual activity and a feedback loop of pain – diminished desire – muscle spasm – pain is easily set in motion. Irregular ovulation and menstrual cycles make conception more difficult and, once pregnant, diabetic women have a higher incidence of miscarriages, stillbirths and abnormal babies. The perinatal mortality rate for babies of diabetic mothers may be as high as 7 times that of non-diabetics (Lion 1982). A diabetic woman who wants to have children, but has difficulty in conceiving or carrying a pregnancy successfully to term and giving birth to a normal infant, may feel that she is failing in her normal female role, and this sense of inadequacy may lower her feelings of self-worth both as a person and as a sexual partner.

Diabetes mellitus is a familial disorder and if one parent is diabetic 25 per cent of children will have the disorder. If both are diabetics the likelihood is that 50 per cent of their offspring will develop diabetes too. Genetic counselling is therefore advisable for diabetics contemplating having a baby, both so that the couple is aware of the facts and to allay what may be unnecessary fears which can themselves inhibit sexual desire and performance.

People with diabetes can have severe emotional reactions related to fear of being disabled, to life-style modifications, and to altered physiological functioning. These emotions in turn can disrupt sexual identity and social relationships as well as sexual relationships. However, it is important to emphasise that well-controlled diabetes mellitus should not disturb usual roles and relationships, and good diabetic control may reduce the likelihood of the kinds of complications that can affect sexual functioning (Woods 1984).

Many other endocrine disturbances can affect sexuality, both by bringing about disordered functioning and by altering physical appearance so that body image, self-concept and self-esteem are prejudiced. Adrenal gland disorders can have both kinds of effect. Undersecretion, or Addison's disease, causes changed skin pigmentation while the oversecretion of Cushing's syndrome alters facial and bodily appearance, possibly producing obesity, hirsutism, acne and purple striae on the abdomen. In women menstruation may be irregular or cease altogether, and men may become impotent.

Overactivity of the thyroid gland leads to physical symptoms such as weight loss, diarrhoea and heart conditions, and to irritability, anxiety and nervousness, which can interrupt sexual self-concept by making the person feel generally unwell and by disturbing relationships with others. Exophthalmos, which may occur with hyperthyroidism, alters facial appearance and may make the person feel ugly and unattractive as a sexual partner. Underactivity of the thyroid gland can also interfere with sexuality both via its general symptoms of fatigue, depression, weight gain and hair loss, and by causing amenorrhoea.

Pituitary hormones, which help control a very wide range of body functions, also influence sexuality in numerous ways. Growth hormone excess or deficit in children will lead to abnormal height and in adults to acromegaly (overgrowth of the hands, feet and lower jaw). Low levels of Thyroid Stimulating Hormone cause thyroid under-activity, with growth retardation in children and symptoms of hypothyroidism in adults. All conditions such as these which affect physical appearance are important for sexuality, because body image and self-concept are highly dependent on presenting an 'appropriate' physique. An 'abnormal' appearance will draw attention to individuals and may cause them and others to evaluate them as unattractive and undesirable companions both socially and sexually.

Dysfunctions of the ovaries or testes are particularly likely to be damaging to self-esteem because, as we saw in Section 1, concepts of femininity and masculinity in our culture are strongly related to reproductive roles. Successful performance of these roles is expected and married couples who do not have children are especially vulnerable to damaged self-esteem and feelings of inadequacy. Infertility will be discussed in more detail later in this chapter in the section on Sexuality and the Reproductive System.

SEXUALITY AND THE ELIMINATORY SYSTEMS

Clients' problems of the eliminatory systems which link with sexuality will be discussed together in this section because many feelings are common to dysfunctions of both urinary and faecal elimination. Social norms and taboos surrounding elimination teach very young children the importance of independence and self-control in managing excretory functions, and notions of cleanliness or dirt and pollution, fastidiousness and privacy which are carefully guarded throughout life. The location of excretory and genital body orifices means that bodily hygiene and sexual matters are closely associated, and sexuality and 'dirtiness' are linked in our moral belief systems too.

People with health problems related to excretion therefore face managing elimination so that their personal hygiene and comfort are maintained and other people are unaware of management activities such as frequent visits to the lavatory, washing soiled linen, and disposing of appliances. Anxiety about 'slipping up' and inadvertently revealing the situation to others may interfere with peace of mind, and this aspect may be much magnified in relation to sexual relationships. People with elimination management problems may feel that they are unclean physically, socially and sexually, and may withdraw from relationships because they cannot imagine others being attracted to them. But if they are involved in intimate relationships, then fear of revealing their situation and of accidents may diminish libido and performance.

All these worries may be present to a varying extent when people have urinary infections, which cause short-term disruptions of sexuality but may lead on to longer-term problems of incontinence, renal failure and stoma formation. Urinary disorders of all kinds are likely to cause fatigue and general feelings of unwellness because of pain or retention of waste products, which means that less physical and emotional energy is available for all kinds of activity, including sexual activity.

Incontinence, both urinary and faecal, pose particular problems for sexual activity because of fear and embarrassment over accidents during intimate relations. Precautions such as plastic sheets or incontinence pads to protect a bed, washing the genital area before having intercourse, and the prospect of explaining the situation to a new partner may banish all thought of sexual activity from the mind, and actual 'disasters' which occur can put a stop to initiatives.

Stoma formation can result in feelings of inadequacy, vulnerability and dirtiness. The external siting of the stoma can cause people to feel abnormal, unattractive and vulnerable to injury, with the result that they may hesitate to see themselves as able to form sexual relationships for a number of reasons. Their body image and self-concept are altered in ways which make it hard to accept that other people may be attracted to them and that sexual activity is possible without damaging the stoma. Depression, anxiety and a diminished self-concept can dampen libido further, and it may take some time for 'ostomates' to adjust to their new body image and gain enough confidence in handling their appliance to be confident that it will remain secure during sexual activity. Stoma formation in itself does not alter physical functioning in ways beyond excretion. Indeed, vitality and sexual feelings may be improved if disabling symptoms such as severe diarrhoea or incontinence are relieved. Fertility remains, normal pregnancy and delivery are the rule, and contraception is a consideration for ostomates.

Incontinence and stoma aids and appliances can seem a major deterrent to physically and psychologically comfortable sexual activity, but in practice seemingly huge problems can be overcome with ingenuity and a down-to-earth approach. Women with indwelling urinary catheters can have vaginal intercourse in the usual way, with the catheter held out of the way and perhaps secured to the abdomen with a small piece of adhesive strapping. A man can bend the catheter along the shaft of the penis and if necessary his partner can use a water-soluble lubricant such as KY jelly to ease penetration. Collecting bags can be disconnected or arranged in an unobtrusive position. Intermittent catheterisation may be an option for some kinds of urinary problems, or manual expression of the bladder before intercourse can minimise the risk of leakage. Because catheterisation is associated with higher rates of urinary infection, careful cleansing of the urinary meatus and catheter are needed by both partners before and after intercourse.

Chronic renal disorders and their treatments, including diet, drugs, dialysis and transplantation, have profound implications for sexuality. Chronic fatigue, weight loss, altered skin colour and many associated symptoms affect self-concept and body image in ways that can lead sufferers to feel inadequate as financial supporters of their familiies, as strong and whole individuals, and as sexual beings. Being unable to keep up paid employment and standards of work at home can lead to crises in self-identity and sexual self-esteem. Severe dietary restrictions limit sensual gratification through eating and detract from the social side of eating with other people. In addition, the specific effects of chronic renal failure include loss of libido for both women and men, and declining fertility due to testicular atrophy or to irregular or absent ovulation. Men may have difficulty in having or maintaining an adequate erection and capacity for orgasm is decreased in both sexes.

Dialysis may bring the possibility of returning to work and resuming a whole range of family and social activities which have had to be dropped, and in this way can make a big contribution to health and sexual expression by restoring self-esteem and a more positive body image. However, some dialysis patients still experience fatigue and say they never feel 'really well'. The dependence on the machine and on other people which accompany dialysis can be undermining because our culture values personal independence and control, which are aspects of gender roles as well as other social roles. Having a 'shunt' or fistula may cause feelings of vulnerability and its appearance may be thought unpleasant to potential sexual partners.

Transplantation too can bring a vast improvement in general quality of life and the kinds of work, home and leisure activities possible. People with transplants, however, may have difficulty in adjusting to their new body image and may feel their new kidney is fragile. This may inhibit them from making the most of their new health potential, including opportunities for sexual encounters. Some post-transplant clients report an improvement in sexual desire and capacity but others have a decline, and all face the possibility of unwanted effects of steroid and anti-hypertensive drugs. Links between sexuality and drug treatments will be discussed in Chapter 7.

In this section, we have seen how problems of elimination are particularly sensitive areas for sexuality because they interfere with the self-concept and body image of wholeness and cleanliness, and this in itself erodes self-esteem. As well as having to cope with these aspects, clients may have to manage appliances which also alter their body image and feelings of attractiveness and desirability. In some cases treatments can add further complications for sexuality.

SEXUALITY AND THE REPRODUCTIVE SYSTEM

Sexual activity is only one aspect of sexuality, but the effects of ill-health on this fundamental facet of human life can be profound. We have seen how sexuality and sexual activity can be compromised by a great number of body dysfunctions and diseases which have complex biopsychosocial effects. Physical, psychological, social and sexual effects of illness are intertwined and problems in each area can have repercussions in the others. But sexual activity in our culture has come to acquire a special status in defining sexuality, and so when illness or dysfunction directly affect the reproductive system, patients' or clients' self-esteem may be threatened to such a high degree that their whole personality and security are challenged.

Sexually-transmitted diseases (STD) are still widely surrounded with moral disapproval despite some relaxation in attitudes in recognition of the fact that sufferers are more likely to seek treatment when this is offered in a non-punitive atmosphere. Nevertheless, many people still connect STD with immorality and loose living, with the result that patients and their contacts feel shame and guilt, and relationships may be destroyed when blame is apportioned. In the short term, sexuality is disrupted by this kind of accusation of deceit, disloyalty and 'promiscuity' because friendships may break up. Additional strain may be caused by the need to suspend sexual activity until treatment is complete and a cure confirmed. In the longer term, STD can have profound implications for sexuality because infertility can result from infected tubes both in women and men, and some recently-highlighted infections such as herpes and AIDS (Acquired Immune Deficiency Syndrome) as yet have no satisfactory treatments. For this reason, people may be advised or may decide for themselves to reduce sexual activity or avoid it altogether so that they do not run the risk of spreading or contacting STD.

A decision to become celibate or use alternative forms of sexual pleasure such as masturbation or non-genital sex may lead to further emotional stress and disrupted relationships. An interesting and relevant question is what is meant by the term 'promiscuity', for excess in any activity is principally a matter of social definition. Alcoholism was once said to be 'drinking more than your doctor', and a parallel definition of promiscuity could be drawn up!

Celibacy is certainly one way to avoid STD but it has its costs, and the development of safe and effective treatments for infections would be more socially and personally satisfactory than moral condemnation as a means of reducing suffering associated with these conditions.

Infertile individuals and couples may experience insecurity over gender identity, but when sexuality is defined in the way we have done in this book it is clear that much more than reproductive ability is included. A person is no less of a woman or man if s/he cannot reproduce, because sexuality involves the total personality and life-style, and not simply procreative and related functions. Nevertheless, social expectations are so great that many people feel they are not completely fulfilled unless they produce their own biological offspring. A mystique has been built up about having one's *own* child which is so great that being a successful social parent by bringing up an adopted child is not an acceptable alternative for many people. An immense amount of anguish and suffering, both emotional and physical, is caused by a diagnosis of infertility and subsequent attempts to treat this. Vast sums of money are also spent by individuals and health services to develop and carry out complex technological manipulations to enable couples to bear children in whose conception and gestation they have played some role, whether through surrogate parenthood (artificial insemination by donor and 'womb-leasing') or in vitro fertilisation and reimplantation of the fertilised ovum.

This is an area where moral debates could be extended from questions of definitions of when life begins and human's rights to create life artificially to those of the morality of a society which imposes such stereotyped definitions of sexuality on its members that they feel compelled to go to these great lengths to become biological parents. In Section 1 we considered evidence for the very powerful effects of socialisation on human development, and suggested that the role of social parent may be more influential than that of biological parent in influencing how children grow up. These considerations inevitably raise questions about whether scarce resources are best spent on expensive 'high-tech' treatments which may benefit very few people and have as yet unknown complications. Spending a similar amount of money on other facilities related to health and sexuality, such as day nurseries and equal opportunities in education and work, would bring benefits to a greater proportion of the population as well as contributing to a redefinition of the very stereotypes which are so personally and socially damaging.

Surgery involving the reproductive system raises related issues for both women and men in a culture where sexual attractiveness and performance are highly rated. Patients undergoing hysterectomy, prostatectomy and sterilisation are often subjected to a barrage of ill-founded tales about the likely effects of these operations. Loss of femininity or masculinity is often said to occur, but these suggestions are based on a very narrow definition of sexuality and inadequate knowledge of the physiological and psychosocial processes underlying sexual activity. Research has shown that the overwhelming majority of women do not feel diminished in any way by hysterectomy or sterilisation. On the contrary, their general health is so much better when they are relieved of distressing and debilitating menstrual symptoms that they are more vigorous and active, and their sex lives may improve. Loss of fertility, far from being a drawback of hysterectomy, comes as a relief to the majority of couples (Webb & Wilson-Barnett 1983). Similarly, with prostatectomy and vasectomy, libido and sexual satisfaction are not imperilled in the vast majority of cases. After prostatectomy by the trans-urethral route libido, erections, orgasm and satisfaction are usually retained, the only adverse effect being retrograde ejaculation with a consequent milky appearance of the urine. Perineal or suprapubic prostatectomy may cause impotence by destroying nervous tissue, but these operations are usually only performed to treat malignant prostatic enlargement. In the case of both female and male surgery of the reproductive tract the best guide to post-operative sexual activity is pre-operative behaviour, and if sex was formerly satisfactory it is likely to remain so after operation. Conversely, surgery is unlikely to bring about sudden improvements in unsatisfactory sexual relationships because it is probable that psychosocial factors play a bigger role than physiological ones where there is sexual dysfunction (Masters & Johnson 1970).

Masters & Johnson followed their research into heterosexual and homosexual behaviour with studies of sexual dysfunction, which had previously been interpreted mainly as a neurotic symptom indicating underlying psychological problems (Masters & Johnson 1970). They were concerned to detect and treat organic factors where these existed, and developed techniques of therapy involving treatment of couples together by a team of two therapists, one a woman and one a man. The couple were treated as a unit, and education about sexual functioning and communication formed the basis for relatively short, intensive treatments.

In women lack of orgasm was the most common dysfunction found by Masters & Johnson and this might be primary, situational, random or secondary anorgasmia. Primary anorgasmia means that orgasm, which is the endpoint release of maximal sexual response, is not reached in any situation. However, orgasm is interpreted differently by individuals and it is first necessary to establish what a woman does feel. When orgasm is experienced in certain circumstances only, this is termed situational anorgasm, while random orgasm may be experienced on an unpredictable basis. Rarely secondary anorgasm happens when someone who previously had orgasms ceases to do so, and this is usually related to an event in life such as death of a partner or ill-health of a physical or psychological nature.

Physical as well as emotional problems can lead to anorgasmia in women, and these include insufficient vaginal lubrication, pain on intercourse (dyspareunia) and chronic pelvic congestion as a result of not achieving release of sexual excitation. Treatment of this, as of many difficulties, begins with removing the pressure to perform and putting an emphasis instead on exploring and communicating the couples' sexual needs, desires and inhibitions. Sexual education is given and specific physical activities are suggested to help the couple give and receive pleasurable stimulation.

Vaginismus is the second commonest dysfunction found in women, and it is an involuntary constriction of the pelvis muscles in the outer third of the vagina and perineum. It is a spastic, reflex response brought about by real, anticipated or imagined attempts at penetration, and most often results from physical or psychological trauma associated with clumsy and inexperienced attempts to have intercourse, or from rape. Strict social norms and prohibitions can also sensitise a woman so that she develops vaginismus.

The diagnosis of vaginismus is made by attempting to perform a vaginal examination using only one finger. This will bring about the involuntary muscle contractions and begin the treatment by showing the couple that it is a truly involuntary condition and not a rejection by the woman of that particular partner. Treatment progresses by the woman and her partner using increasingly larger dilators until finally she is able to have intercourse. Dyspareunia is a common cause of vaginismus and may result from vaginal infection, allergic reactions to products such as soap or vaginal deodorants, or douching. Ceasing to use the product or douches, which are unnecessary for personal hygiene in any case, will cure the discomfort. Vaginal dryness when lubrication diminishes at the menopause can be treated by using a lubricant such as KY jelly or an oestrogen cream.

Masters & Johnson's treatments always involve couples. More recently, women have formed pre-orgasmic groups of approximately six women who meet regularly to share their difficulties and feelings, and to give each other information and support. The groups are called 'pre-orgasmic' because their members believe that everyone is capable of having orgasms, and after group meetings women do 'homework' exercises involving progressive self-stimulation to learn about their own feelings and sensations. After achieving orgasm by masturbation, partners are involved in homework assignments if the individual women wish. The advantages of these groups are that participants are able to learn to understand how their bodies work and that people help themselves rather than relying on professionals whose services may be expensive or not easily available. Unlike Masters & Johnson's therapy, these groups are not restricted to married couples and therefore single or homosexual people can seek help from them.

Impotence, or inability to achieve or maintain an erection, is the most common sexual dysfunction found in men. Those who have never had a sufficient erection to achieve intercourse are said to have primary impotence, and the causes are similar to those of vaginismus in women, namely traumatic and/or unsuccessful attempts at intercourse or strong prohibitive social mores. The problem becomes compounded by 'performance anxiety'. Secondary impotence develops after some successful experience of intercourse and may be due to excess alcohol intake or premature ejaculation. As for female dysfunctions, treatment involves removing the pressure to perform and teaching couples 'sensate focus' exercises through which they learn to stimulate each other without penetration and intercourse. They are encouraged to communicate their needs verbally or non-verbally, to indicate what gives them pleasure, and to discuss any fears they may have.

Disorders of ejaculation are the second commonest group of problems found in men. Premature ejaculation is defined by Masters & Johnson (1970) as present when in at least 50 per cent of occasions ejaculation happens before the partner is satisfied. This may be a result of performance anxiety, the man feeling the need to demonstrate that he can ejaculate adequately. Distraction techniques to divert attention from ejaculation and decrease anxiety are not usually effective because they may reduce stimulation so that erection is lost. As before, counselling and communication between couples are the basis of treatment, and in addition 'squeeze' techniques may be helpful. The method recommended by Masters & Johnson is for the partner to stimulate the penis by hand, and when the man has reached the plateau phase (see Chapter 1), to place the thumb on the frenulum of the penis and the first two fingers of the hand above and below the glans. Squeezing with enough pressure for the man to feel, but not to cause discomfort, will then prevent ejaculation and by this form of 'reconditioning' greater ejaculatory control should be achieved.

Other dysfunctions of ejaculation include ejaculatory incompetence, when the man is unable to ejaculate with the penis in the vagina. A check for congenital absence of the ejaculatory ducts should be done, but, for those who can ejaculate, training exercises of a similar kind to those already described may be used. Retrograde ejaculation, or ejaculation into the bladder and not via the urethra, may be caused by surgery such as prostatectomy or by various medical conditions including diabetes and spinal cord injury.

Masters & Johnson's pioneering treatments of sexual dysfunctions form the basis for present day sex therapy. They build on the premises that physiological sex acts are similar in women and men, and that dysfunctions result most commonly from double standards for women and men, unrealistic expectations, fear of failure, and poor communications between couples of their needs and what they find pleasurable.

CONCLUSION

In this chapter we have discussed how illnesses and body dys-functions can affect sexuality via the threats they pose to self-.concept, body image and feelings of self-worth. These effects are complex because biological, psychological, social and sexual causes and effects are inseparable and reinforce each other. What starts out as a physiological disturbance, like a heart attack for instance, can rapidly go on to produce psychosocial and sexual complications. Similarly, a condition which affects the sexual organs, such as infection, can have repercussions for other phy-siological functions, psychological state and social relationships. Treatments for diseases and dysfunctions can add to the problems, as we saw in the specific cases of surgery and dialysis as well as in the general implications of becoming a patient or entering hospit-al. Drug treatments are another factor which can either promote or impair health and sexuality, and it is to these that we turn in the next chapter.

CHAPTER 7

Drugs and Sexuality

Probably no medical treatment has purely positive effects on the body. The involvement of sexuality in adverse results of hospitalisation, with its deprivations of independence, control and privacy, surgery and its erosion of concepts of wholeness and body integrity, and renal dialysis and its accompanying machine-dependence and dietary restrictions have featured in earlier chapters. Drugs are another type of treatment which can have both positive and negative influences on sexuality and sexual performance, whether substances are used for 'recreational' or 'therapeutic' reasons.

A drug which improves health by relieving or curing distressing or disabling symptoms will increase feelings of well-being and improve quality of life. Greater physical and emotional vigour and energy will repair damaged self-esteem, enable recovered patients to resume family and work responsibilities and enjoy social life again, and along with these enhancements sexual self-concept will be restored and libido regained. Depression and lethargy resulting from the illness will be eased and the person will again become interested in and able to participate in social activities, including sexual acts.

Unwanted effects of drugs, however, have the opposite effect. General, non-life threatening side-effects may in reality be very disruptive to quality of life by reducing feelings of energy and well-being and by causing depression, with lethargy, social withdrawal and loss of interest in personal appearance. Gastrointestinal disturbances are common side-effects of a wide range of drugs including digoxin, diuretics and iron preparations. Nausea, vomiting, and diarrhoea are all very debilitating and unpleasant symptoms which sap energy and distract their sufferers from enjoying life. They may cut a person off from social and sexual encounters and thus add depression and isolation to existing symptoms. Skin reactions too are common drug reactions, and their unsightliness may make the sufferer and others less interested in close relationships of all kinds, including sexual relations, because notions of attractiveness and desirability are so entwined with physical appearance.

Specific effects on sexual functioning also occur with many drugs, and if takers are unaware of the possibility of their sexual feelings or performance being affected they may become confused and depressed about their altered sexual responses. Individuals vary greatly in their physiological and psychological make-up and it is impossible to predict accurately how a person may respond to any drug, including its effects on sexuality. More is known about the effects of drugs on men's sexual functioning because more research has been carried out and this difference is probably related to two factors. First, disordered function in men is readily observed because erection is required for sexual intercourse and because men are expected to have an orgasm with every sexual encounter. In women, however, the signs are less prominent, and women are not expected to have an orgasm at every, or even the majority of, sexual encounters. Secondly, the majority of scientists have been, and continue to be, male and this will condition the kinds of topics they find interesting and satisfying to study (Birke *et al* 1980).

Nevertheless, information exists about the undesired effects of many drugs on sexual functioning, and it is likely that this represents the small, visible portion of a 'submerged iceberg' of other effects which will be revealed as more research is done. In this chapter we shall examine the unwanted side-effects on sexuality which accompany common drugs used for 'recreational' and 'therapeutic' reasons, and which are summarised in Figures 7.1 and 7.2 at the end of the chapter.

RECREATIONAL DRUGS

Recreational drugs, whether legal or illegal, are used to produce relaxation and pleasant sensations. Sometimes their takers also hope for aphrodisiac effects which will improve libido and sexual satisfaction, but the results often turn out to be quite the reverse.

Alcohol is the commonest recreational drug in the West and, contrary to what many people believe, it has a negative effect on sexual functioning. Initially, it produces relaxation, relieves social inhibitions and increases sexual desire, but its central nervous system depressant action rapidly intervenes and inhibits actual performance. Additionally, its diuretic effect can disrupt sexual activity! The destructive results of alcohol use, particularly in the long-term, outweigh its doubtful short-term benefits because the changes it brings can lead to violence, broken relationships and inadequate functioning in work, family and social life. Domestic violence is frequently associated with alcohol abuse and the majority of rapes take place under the influence of alcohol (Brown-miller 1976). The specific long-term complications of alcohol for sexual functioning are decreased libido, impotence and difficulty in achieving orgasm. Ultimately, sterility results and men develop gynaecomastia. When these associations with alcohol use are considered, it might seem surprising that it is still a legal subst-ance, especially in view of the moral indignation surrounding the illegal drug cannabis or marijuana. This contradiction shows that rules about legality or illegality are questions of social definition at particular moments in history rather than the results of a scientific balancing of evidence. If alcohol and nicotine were drugs being evaluated for safety prior to legal release today, they would probably never be permitted to circulate so widely because their unwanted effects are so dangerous and extensive.

Smoke containing *nicotine* constricts blood vessels and has the effect of reducing pulmonary capacity, with cough and shortness of breath on exercise. Thus, the amount of exertion possible during sexual acts is reduced and foul-smelling breath and coughing, which are inevitable consequences of cigarette smok-ing, may make users unattractive as sexual partners. Women smokers have more miscarriages, stillbirths and small-for-gestational-age babies, and men's sperm production decreases both in quantity and mobility (Woods 1984).

Marijuana (cannabis) use is often linked with sexual 'permissive-ness' but, although its users may claim it has enhancing effects, it is in fact a central nervous system depressant. Like alcohol, it starts by freeing inhibitions and producing relaxation, and also height-ens sensations, produces warm and affectionate feelings, and alters perceptions of time. Therefore subjective pleasure is greater and apparently longer lasting, but decreased libido and potency are more likely with higher doses and longer use. A notable difference between alcohol and marijuana use is that lethargy rather than violence and aggression occur with marijuana. Some of the enhancing effects claimed for marijuana may be more related to the social setting and company in which it used, rather than its pharmacological effects, for users tend to be more non-traditional in their attitudes than the general population (Hogan 1980, Weinberg 1982).

Opiates, including *cocaine, sedatives, tranquillisers and hypnotics* all have a depressant effect on the central nervous system, so that initial relaxation and freeing of inhibitions is replaced by reductions in sexual drive and capability. In men, impotence and ejaculatory failure are found and the sperm count may be reduced. Women users may suffer from dysmenorrhoea, amenorrhoea, reduced fertility and an increased rate of spontaneous abortions. These substances also have a profoundly disruptive effect on work, family and social life such that financial independence may be lost, interpersonal relationships are destroyed, and a sense of worth in the view of self and others is diminished, adding to feelings of inadequacy due to failure in sexual activities.

'Uppers' or *stimulating drugs* of various kinds are reputed to have aphrodisiac effects but they probably have little or no influence on libido and sexual performance beyond subjective impressions. They may enhance enjoyment for users but partners will not observe any objective 'improvement' in capacity. Amphetamine and cocaine relieve fatigue and heighten moods, so that sexual activity can occur when previously the individual was too tired, and orgasmic sensations may be improved. Alternatively, a state of agitation is produced that prevents focussed activity, including sexual acts. Cocaine has variously been said to cause spontaneous erections and multiple orgasms, or prolonged painful erections (priapism). Hallucinogenic substances such as LSD (lysergic acid diethylamide) and 'angel dust' (mescaline phencyclidine) alter perceptions and produce extravagant mental images, loss of inhibitions and prolonged sensations of orgasms. However, the impressions created may be so diverting that they distract attention and concentration and so render sexual activity impossible.

Recreational drugs, whether legal or illegal, are remarkably similar in their effects on sexuality. In small doses or for short-term use they may improve sexual desire and enjoyment by bringing about a state of relaxation and disinhibition. Progressively, however, they have a depressant or distracting effect which interferes not only with sexual performance but also with all other aspects of life, so that usual social functioning is no longer possible, personal and intimate relationships break up, and mental health suffers. Judgements about the relative merits, morality and legal desirability of particular substances are based on personal values and historical accidents rather than systematic investigation and rational judgement. The ideal recreational or aphrodisiac drug does not exist and perhaps never will, because many centuries have already been devoted to the search and have met with no success.

THERAPEUTIC DRUGS

Antidepressant drugs can play a positive role in sexual expression by elevating moods and bringing about an increase in interests and activities, including sexual activity. However, the mechanism of action of some of these agents results in negative effects on sexual functioning which can counterbalance or even outweigh their positive effects.

Tricyclic antidepressants such amitriptyline and imipramine have anticholinergic actions and can cause impotence and ejaculatory difficulties, and both sexes may experience delay in reaching orgasm. Mono amine oxidase inhibitors, of which phenelzine and tranylcypromine are examples, can have similar effects. Some sexual difficulties have been reported with lithium carbonate, but research has not yet confirmed the nature and extent of these (Woods 1984). Sedative effects produced by some anti-depressants can dampen energy and interest levels for all kinds of activities and this would be detrimental to sexual functioning as well as to role performance, and interest taken in appearance and social activities.

Antihistamines like diphenhydramine, chlorpheniramine and promethazine are used mainly to control symptoms of allergic reactions in the form of hay fever and itching. These symptoms are uncomfortable for the sufferer and possibly aesthetically unpleasant for other people, and as such can be disruptive of social life and make the individual feel unattractive as a companion and as a sexual partner. Suppression of symptoms can therefore contribute to enhanced feelings of well-being and improved self-esteem by restoring the body image to a pleasant one. At the same time, the blocking of parasympathetic nerve impulses to the sex organs produced by antihistamines can cause decreased vaginal lubrication in women and impotence in men. Drowsiness can also reduce sexual interest.

Antihypertensives are a widely used group of drugs frequently associated with sexual dysfunction, but the picture is complicated by the fact that patients with hypertension may have sexual dysfunctions as part of the disease process too. They may lead stressful lives, which can reduce sexual drive, and may have cardiovascular symptoms such as angina and heart failure which will interfere with sexual function. Nevertheless, the peripheral sympathetic blocking action of propranolol, reserpine, methyldopa and clonidine can lead to drowsiness which reduces libido and even to depression, with its dampening of interest and energy for a whole range of activities including sexual activity. Specific effects on sexual functioning include impotence and retrograde ejaculation in men, and difficulty in having an orgasm in women.

Diuretic drugs can also have effects on sexual functioning, but the way this occurs is not well understood. Possibly potassium depletion is a factor in loss of libido. Women taking diuretics such as chlorothiazide or bendrofluazide may experience amenorrhoea and breast soreness, while men may have impotence or gynaecomastia. Spironolactone, although acting in a different way by displacing aldosterone in the kidneys, can also cause similar difficulties. The fact that antihypertensives and diuretics may be taken in combination increases the possibility of sexual dysfunction resulting.

Antispasmodic drugs are used to relax smooth muscle in the digestive, biliary and urinary tracts, and propantheline is the most widely used example. It can cause decreased libido for both sexes, and decreased vaginal lubrication in women and impotence in men via its anti-cholinergic effects.

Cytoxic drugs are used to destroy malignant cells or prevent their proliferation, and their action is greater on cells which divide more rapidly. For this reason they interfere with sperm production and cause temporary sterility in men, and women may experience amenorrhoea. Nausea, vomiting, diarrhoea, severe tiredness and general feelings of unwellness accompany administration of many cytotoxic substances, including cyclophosphamide, methotrexate, fluorouracil and actinomycin D. Some substances cause alopecia which, together with other distressing side-effects and the devastating implications of knowing that one has a malignant disease, can be profoundly detrimental to body image and self-concept. Patients may feel that they are no longer whole, that the disease process is attacking their body integrity, and that their physical appearance is ugly if they have lost a lot of weight. All these factors will interrupt normal activities of living, and personal and intimate relationships and sexual desire may suffer in the process. Women experiencing amenorrhoea may feel that, on top of everything else, their femininity is reduced by loss of this sign that their bodies are working normally. The effects of radiotherapy on physical, psychological and sexual functions are very similar to those of cytotoxic drugs.

Corticosteroid drugs may be used to treat malignant conditions, and patients may therefore have to contend with their side-effects as well as those of other medications. Drugs like prednisone and prednisolone are used in a wide range of other situations too, and asthma, arthritis, Crohn's disease and ulcerative colitis are some of the most common of these. Specific effects on sexual functioning include decreased libido in both sexes, and in men the sperm count may be reduced and impotence can occur. The generalised side-effects of steroid use can also have important consequences for sexuality. Mood changes may occur, ranging from enhanced feelings of well-being to depression, with its suppressant effects on libido and on social and sexual activities. Changes in physical appearance can disturb body image and lower self-esteem in people who experience weight gain and alterations in body shape and facial appearance, acquiring a 'moon face' and perhaps skin pigmentation, acne and purple striae on the abdomen. All these effects, together with the symptoms of the serious conditions treated by steroid administration and the possible side-effects of other medications being taken simultaneously, are likely to affect sexuality in important ways.

Oral contraceptives are another group of substances which can have both positive and negative effects on sexuality. Freedom from constant fears of unwanted pregnancy can be life-enhancing in many areas, lifting depression and enabling women to take more active roles in work, family, social and sexual spheres. The relief from dysmenorrhoea, pre-menstrual tension, irregular or heavy menstrual bleeding that comes with taking the pill can be very beneficial. Whilst libido is improved for some women once these problems are removed, others experience depression and a decrease in sexual desire. Other possible side-effects like nausea, headache, lethargy, breast discomfort or fluid retention may reduce interest and energy levels so that sexual activity is less desired. A few women develop a 'butterfly-mask' of facial pigmentation (chloasma) and some contact lens wearers are unable to tolerate wearing their lenses while taking the pill; in either of these cases, women may judge their physical and sexual attractiveness to be marred as an indirect result of taking oral contraceptives. Changing to a different preparation with different doses or combinations of hormones may reduce side-effects, but for some women these irritating and debilitating problems, while not dangerous to health, will make the pill unacceptable.

The implications for sexuality of taking *sedatives, hypnotics and tranquillisers* such as the benzodiazepines (diazepam, lorazepam, chlordiazepoxide, and so on), phenothiazides (chlorpromazine, thioridazine and prochlorperazine), meprobromate and methaqualone are the same when these substances are taken therapeutically as when they are taken recreationally, as discussed earlier in this chapter. Relaxation and freeing of inhibitions may have some beneficial effects, but decreased libido, impotence and ejaculatory failure can occur.

Miscellaneous drugs in common use which affect sexuality are L-dopa and cimetidine. The improvement in symptoms of Parkinson's disease which results from taking L-dopa probably accounts for any increase in sexual activity. The patient feels generally well, and quality of life and all-round enjoyment are regained, the sexual sphere being just one of several areas of improvement. The occurrence of specific sexual rejuvenating effects have not been proved. With cimetidine, temporary impotence has been reported (Woods 1984).

Polypharmacy, or the simultaneous prescription of a number of medications, is widespread in Western medicine. Chronic cardiovascular, renal and respiratory dysfunctions are notable examples of conditions treated by polypharmacy. Patients with angina, hypertension and mild heart failure may be taking antihypertensive, diuretic and tranquillising drugs together. A steroid may be given if these patients also have arthritis, and many drug-takers will also add cigarettes or alcohol to their list.

The elderly are a group who are particularly likely to be subject to polypharmacy, with its attendant opportunities for unwanted side-effects of all kinds including effects on sexuality. The myth that elderly people lose interest in sexuality and sexual activity leads to a lack of consideration of the needs of elderly people, and the possibly deleterious effects of drugs on these aspects of their lives are ignored.

TYPE OF DRUG	MODE OF ACTION	EFFECT ON SEXUALITY
Alcohol	CNS depressant, diuretic	Short term: relaxation, freeing of inhibitions Long term: decreased libido, orgasmic dysfunction, sterility Men: impotence, gynaecomastia
Amphetamines and cocaine	CNS stimulants	Relief of fatigue, heightened moods, delayed orgasm Men: delayed ejaculation High doses: loss of libido, distracting agitation Women: vaginal dryness Men: impotence
Hallucinogens	Altered perceptions	Relaxation, freeing of inhibitions, enhanced subjective sensations, possibly decreased libido and performance due to distracting thoughts
Marijuana	CNS depressant	Relaxation, freeing of inhibitions, increased suggestibility and sensations, increased subjective pleasure Long term or high doses: decreased libido Men: decreased potency decreased sperm count
Nicotine	Vasoconstriction, reduced blood oxygen levels	Breathlessness on exertion, halitosis, cough Women: increased incidence of miscarriage, stillbirth, small-for-gestational-age babies Men: decreased sperm count and mobility
Sedatives, tranquillisers, hypnotics	CNS depressant, blocking of ANS transmission, suppression of pituitary function	Relaxation, freeing of inhibitions, decreased libido Men: impotence, ejaculatory failure

Key CNS = Central Nervous System
ANS = Autonomic Nervous System

Figure 7.1 Summary of effects of 'recreational' drugs on sexuality

TYPE OF DRUG	MODE OF ACTION	EFFECT ON SEXUALITY
Antidepressants	CNS depression, blocking of sympathetic transmission affecting innervation of sex organs	Relief of depression. Tricyclics: delayed orgasm Men: impotence, ejaculatory dysfunction Mono Amine Oxidase Inhibitors: delay or absence of orgasm Men: impotence
Antihistamines	Blocking of parasympathetic transmission causing vasoconstriction in sex organs, CNS depression	Sedation causing decreased libido Women: decreased vaginal lubrication Men: impotence
Antihypertensives	Blocking of sympathetic transmission to sex organs	Depression, sedation causing decreased libido Men: impotence, retrograde ejaculation
Cortico-steroids	Anti-androgenic	Altered appearance: weight gain, skin pigmentation, acne, purple striae Decreased libido Men: reduced sperm count, impotence

Figure 7.2 Summary of effects of 'therapeutic' drugs on sexuality

Furthermore, general pharmacology textbooks do not usually focus attention on the effects of drugs on sexuality and sexual functioning, and a specialist text on sexuality needs to be consulted to acquire this information.

CONCLUSION

It is possible that many drugs have implications for sexuality of which we are unaware, and so a proportion of undesirable effects may go unnoticed. Patients might be able to adjust to side-effects if they understood them and considered the beneficial effects of their medications to outweigh the negative aspects. Others might

TYPE OF DRUG	MODE OF ACTION	EFFECT ON SEXUALITY
Cytotoxics	Destroy cells or prevent cell multiplication	Fatigue, malaise, nausea, depression, alopecia Women: amenorrhoea Men: decreased sperm count
Diuretics	Increased excretion of water, sodium, and possibly potassium via the kidneys	Loss of libido Women: amenorrhoea, breast soreness Men: impotence, gynaecomastia
Oral contraceptives	Suppression of hormone production, prevention of implantation of fertilised ovum	Relieves anxiety about unwanted pregnancy, regular menstrual cycle, relief of dysmenorrhoea. Possibly decreased libido, nausea, headaches, breast soreness, irritability, weight gain, moniliasis (thrush), chloasma (facial pigmentation), post-pill amenorrhoea
Sedatives, tranquillisers, hypnotics	CNS depressants, blocking of ANS transmission, suppression of pituitary function	Relaxation, freeing of inhibitions, decreased libido Men: impotence, ejaculatory failure

Key CNS = Central Nervous System
      ANS = Autonomic Nervous System

decide that the treatment was worse than the disease, and choose to stop their drugs or ask for an alternative prescription. Lack of information about possible side-effects of all kinds can be not only dangerous, if potentially serious complications are ignored, but also very distressing. Loss of libido, impotence, vaginal dryness or delayed orgasm are likely to undermine self-esteem and concepts of personal and social competence and worth whatever the cause, but these effects might be lessened if patients were aware that the changes were drug-induced and would, in the majority of cases, disappear when the medication was stopped. Greater knowledge about the undesirable effects of drugs on sexuality is needed by professionals and clients alike if a truly holistic approach to care is to become a reality.

CHAPTER 8

Sexuality and Carers in the Community

Community care can be cheaper than institutional care as well as offering a higher quality of life, for people want to maintain their dignity and independence and families often wish to take care of elderly parents or relatives who took care of them when they were young. The proportion of elderly people in the population is rising and the majority continue to live in the community, either independently or with their families. There are three times as many disabled people being cared for at home compared with institutional care (Townsend 1981) and there are probably more women caring for elderly and handicapped dependents than there are looking after children under 16 (Oliver 1983). On the other hand, male carers in the community are a minority and are more likely to be the husbands of elderly women and to be retired themselves.

Sexuality and community care are closely related in several ways. The assumption that women are the 'natural' carers, backed up by beliefs that the majority of women do not work outside the home but are full-time housewives, leads many people to conclude that not only children and healthy adult men but also the sick and disabled should be cared for at home by women. In reality, 40 per cent of married women aged between 20 and 40 are in paid employment, at a time when childrearing activities are at a peak, and for those in the 40 to 60 age group the figure rises to approximately 70 per cent (Department of Employment 1981). Personal identity is highly related to feelings of independence and personal worth which come from the social roles we play, and people who have to give up an important role will suffer a blow to their self-esteem which in itself can cause doubts about femininity or masculinity. It is well-documented, too, that being isolated at home or losing one's job can lead to depression, with its negative consequences for sexual interest and performance (Brown & Harris 1978; Gore 1978). Loss of independence and earnings mean that opportunities to travel, go to the cinema or have a meal out are cut. There is less money to spend on personal items like clothes and hairdressing, so people feel less and less like seeking opportunities for social activities, and their chances of meeting a possible sexual partner or forming a close, confiding relationship are greatly diminished. Health may suffer as a result of the physical and emotional burden of caring, because it is difficult to find time to visit the doctor or dentist, or have a much-needed treatment. It is through all these multiple and complex inter-relationships that caring in the community can have effects on self-esteem, body image and sexual life.

WHO CARES?

The unmarried daughter caring for elderly parents has now been replaced by the married woman who works at least part-time and also has her own family to look after. The majority of women today marry and their lives become a cycle of caring which begins when they have children, continues into a phase of looking after elderly parents, and ends with responsibility for a sick and ageing husband, for most marriages involve a woman who is younger than her spouse. Women have a longer life expectancy than men, which results in a greater number of widowed, elderly women needing care, and this is usually given by another woman. Women carers who are not related to the elderly woman they care for are found in greater numbers than men caring for a non-relative, but only 11 per cent of carers for the elderly are not relatives (Equal Opportunities Commission 1981).

WHO HELPS?

Community care philosophies are based on the belief that many people in the community are involved in caring for the sick, disabled and elderly, but studies of who does the caring disprove this. Levels of help from neighbours are low and focus not on major areas of responsibility and routine or heavier tasks like feeding, washing and laundry, but on peripheral or casual assistance with shopping and transport (Equal Opportunities Commission 1984). The amount and kinds of help women carers receive from other family members is similary limited, which means that women may have three jobs. They care for a sick or dependent relative, run the home, and work at an outside job. Male carers usually receive more help from friends, neighbours and relatives, probably because men are not expected in our culture to have to, or be able to, do housework, cooking and laundry. The Equal Opportunities Commission (EOC) report on *Carers and Services* (EOC 1984) showed that 54 per cent of male carers were helped with laundry by relatives, friends and neighbours, compared with 19 per cent of women carers. Similarly, 44 per cent of men but only 29 per cent of women received help with shopping, and 21 per cent were aided with housework compared with 12 per cent of women.

Social service assistance too should be a cornerstone of community care if the quality of life of clients and carers is to be maintained (Opit 1978). However, in a study of the experience of caring, the EOC (1980) reported that only 14 per cent of households with an informal carer received free home help services, 3 per cent received meals on wheels regularly, and 3 per cent did so occasionally or were on a waiting list. Not all areas have a laundry service for incontinent clients and, even where this exists, a waiting list may in effect ration the assistance (Opit 1978).

The kind of formal assistance received by female and male carers also differs both in amount and in its pattern. Male carers are helped more by social services both with domestic tasks and personal care (EOC 1984). Forty-nine per cent of men received help with housework, compared with 28 per cent of women, and 31 per cent of men had cooking assistance while 11 per cent of women received this in a study of community care in a part of the country where provisions were at a fairly high level relative to other areas. Similarly, 29 per cent of male carers but only 10 per cent of women had social service help with toileting the dependent person, and 40 per cent of men were assisted with washing compared with 8 per cent of women. This suggests that male carers are more likely to receive the kind of help that enables them to carry on working full-time with little or no incursion of caring into their working lives. Women, on the other hand, are more likely to give up work entirely or change from a full-time to a part-time job so that they can fulfill the caring role which is expected of them. They struggle to do this with little formal and informal help until their own health is at risk, when short-term relief is given to them. The EOC study (1984) showed that women carers are more likely than men to receive day care or short-stay care for their dependent, and this seems to indicate that women were not offered help or did not seek it until their situation became intolerable, because they and others expected them to cope. Crisis intervention then aimed at giving them a short respite so that they could resume their former caring role whereas if, like male carers, they had received more support earlier a crisis might have been prevented.

Carers are critical, too, of lack of assistance when people are discharged from hospital. Notice that the patient can come home may be given in a telephone call or at visiting time, when a nurse or doctor says that the carer can take the patient home immediately. There is thus no time to prepare the home by getting aids and equipment, food, clean laundry and so on ready, nor for the carer to prepare psychologically and arrange for family and friends to help. Instructions and advice about care at home may not be given, and promised social services may not materialise due to administrative inefficiency (Simpson & Levitt 1981; Finch & Groves 1984).

Caring for a handicapped or sick child is a completely different matter from bringing up a healthy daughter or son. The expected growing independence of the child and resulting freedom from responsibility, particularly for the mother, do not materialise. Instead, as the child grows bigger, caring tasks become heavier and possibly more embarrassing and unpleasant for child and parent alike. Whereas the majority of women with children carry on or resume work at least part-time, the mother of a handicapped child may be unable to do so. The rewards of bringing up a child successfully, seeing personality development and growing independence, may be replaced by a wearing, unending routine accompanied by feelings of guilt, failure, regret and desperation.

All carers in the community, then, bear a burden of extra work with less than optimal assistance from social services, relatives, friends and family. The kinds of tasks involved are repetitive, heavy and unrewarding because there is little to show for all the labour of washing, cleaning and cooking. As soon as the work is done, it gets undone and the round begins again. Studies of housework in general and of informal caring report that those involved, who are in the vast majority of cases women, suffer from feelings of isolation, meaninglessness and lack of control in their lives (Oakley 1974; Finch & Groves 1984). Depression is more common when people are confined to the home, and carers have a reduced quality of life in many areas, including relationships with the person cared for, sexuality in general and their sex lives in particular.

RELATIONSHIPS AND CARING

Many people want to take care of their relatives and friends when they become sick, disabled or elderly and they gain immense personal satisfaction from doing so. In return, their relationship with the dependent person grows richer and a deeper understanding develops in the process of giving and receiving care.

In other situations, however, the enforced mutual loss of independence involved in caring damages or destroys what has previously been a worthwhile and rewarding relationship. Both parties may resent the loss of freedom of privacy, and doing intimate tasks like attending to an incontinent person can be so embarrassing that tempers become frayed and tolerance cannot be kept up. Carers are obliged to perform, and dependents to receive, care which goes against usual norms of modesty between relatives. It is more likely to be a daughter-in-law who cares for her husband's father, for instance, than the son himself. Married couples, too, do not necessarily become comfortable with the intimate aspects of carrying out personal hygiene, and both can feel that they have suffered a loss of dignity.

Dependent people may react in a variety of ways to their enforced circumstances, and this in itself can make additional emotional demands of the carer. Some dependents are afraid to be left alone in case they fall or need something which they cannot get for themselves. Others may feel insecure when left alone even when their physical needs are met. Carers may therefore even have difficulty finding time to be alone in a separate room of the house, to take a bath or wash their hair, to make a relaxed telephone call, or to entertain visitors in privacy. It may be very hard to arrange opportunities to leave the house to go shopping, meet friends and join in social activities, or even to visit the doctor or dentist, and a 'sitter' may not be easily accepted by the dependent even if one is available.

Sick, handicapped or disabled persons too may be deprived of the privacy most of us expect at least in some aspects of life. They may share a bedroom or be confined to one room in which all activities have to be carried out, from eating and entertaining to using a commode or being attended to after an episode of incontinence. Sometimes that room may be one which others use as a living room if the house is crowded or a bed is brought into a living room to provide company and stimulation for the dependent person.

Independence in choosing our clothing and the way we style our hair is something we normally take for granted, but for both carers and dependents this is another side of life which may have to change. Less money may be available for clothes if either or both partners in the caring relationship has had to give up or cut down on paid work, and spend extra money on equipment, supplies or special food. But even if money is available, the opportunity to go out, gain access to shops and fitting rooms, choose and buy clothes or visit a hairdresser may be impossible or very difficult to arrange. Dependent people may be entirely subject to their carers' choice of clothing and may need carers to cut and style their hair. When this is done in a well-meaning but unskilled way, the results can be distressing and disruptive to body image and self-esteem. Dependents may be so grateful to have services done that they do not like to criticise or appear demanding, or alternatively may show their anger and hurt carers' feelings. Carers can also be severely limited by the demands of caring and lack of help, so that they too are unable to keep up their former standards of dress and appearance, and then may feel demoralised and unwilling to take up the few chances for socialising which may present themselves.

Emotional blackmail is a response by dependents which carers find particularly hard to cope with because it brings out feelings of guilt about their own health and independence compared with that of their dependent. Guilt is a reaction women carers are particularly likely to have because they have been taught that caring is their responsibility, and they are very vulnerable to suggestions of failure because caring is tied in with definitions of femininity in our culture. Therefore if a woman feels she is failing as a carer, she may also feel herself to be a failure as a woman, and her dependent and others may deliberately or inadvertently reinforce this notion. Comments such as 'He knows I cannot bear to see him cry so I just give in and do what he wants' are frequently made to researchers (Oliver 1984). Strained tempers and emotional exhaustion can interfere also with carers' relationships with their own partners and children, with jealousy and accusations of neglect if undue attention is felt to be given to the dependent person. Another situation which can arise is that where 'When I am with him, he expects me to do everything for him – turn the TV on, make drinks, help him round the house. But when I have to go out, I come back to find he has managed all these things by himself' (Oliver 1984). When the strains of caring and being cared for reduce relatives to such levels of manipulation, what was previously a labour of love degenerates into an inescapable nightmare of mutual dependence and desperation, but 'the labour must continue even where the love falters' (Graham 1984).

THE COSTS OF CARING

The kind of community care we have at present is certainly cheaper than institutional care, so long as costs are measured in financial terms for the welfare state (Rimmer 1984). In response to claims by social scientists like Goffman (1968) in his book *Asylums* that all institutions are bad, to government policies of cutting public expenditure, and to complaints by patients and clients of the depersonalising effects of 'conveyor belt' treatment, long-stay psychiatric institutions are being closed down and hospital stays are growing ever shorter. Cost-benefit analyses, however, take no account of the hidden costs for informal carers and particularly for women.

Reduced costs for the welfare state are achieved because 'hotel' services – food, hygiene, laundry – and associated staffing costs are borne by individuals and their carers instead of the state. Social security benefits are intended to compensate to some extent for increased personal expenditure, but they do not approach adequate levels. Services like home helps and meals on wheels are limited in availability, and untrained volunteers receiving only reimbursement of their expenses are used to substitute trained professionals (Thomas 1984). Using devices such as these, community care becomes the cheap option it could not be if social services were provided at a level matching needs, with no waiting lists or rationing, widespread and free provision of facilities and equipment such as laundry services, continence and mobility aids, and adequate levels of benefits to compensate for loss of earnings and the additional expenses involved in caring.

Carers who give up or reduce their paid work suffer not only an immediate reduction in income, but also possible longer-term financial loss. The size of an occupational pension is based on the number of years when contributions were paid and the salary

level, so that those leaving work early have their pension calculated on fewer years and lower salary levels. They may even lose
their pension rights altogether. Going part-time or having a break
in employment to become a carer will have detrimental effects on
career development and promotion prospects in the same way as
they do for married women who take time out to bring up
children.

Social security benefits, in addition to not being high enough to
compensate for lost earnings, are sometimes paid in a discrimina-
tory way. Most advisory leaflets address themselves to househol-
ders as men, saying for example, 'If you or you and your wife
between you have savings. . .' or 'You may need extra benefit. . . for
yourself, your wife or for your children', which is inappropriate
for a society in which 10 per cent of households are headed by
single parents and only 30 per cent consist of a married couple
living with their dependent children. Material discrimination
exists in the restriction of Invalid Care Allowance to men and
single women, and the fact that women can only claim Non-
contributory Invalidity Pension if they are unable to do 'normal
household duties'. These regulations are based on the idea that it
is 'natural' for married women to stay at home and not earn
money, and that housework is a normal activity for women but not
for men. They demonstrate the kind of biological reductionist
thinking that we criticised in Section 1.

As a result of the almost inevitable fall in income suffered by
carers, together with the extra expenses involved in caring for a
sick or dependent person, carers' standard of living is likely to be
reduced. New clothes, social activities and holidays may be
impossible to afford even if the caring role permits them. Furniture and home decorations may wear out or be spoiled more
quickly as a result of the use of a wheelchair or other equipment
like calipers, which rub against upholstery or bed linen. More
frequent laundering of linen for incontinent people makes its life
shorter, special food or clothing may be required, or extra transport costs incurred if a dependent is unable to use public transport.

The emotional strain of caring can be extremely wearing, because
of its constant nature and the fact that there is no end in sight.
Carers may take on the role expecting it to last a short time, but
then find themselves committed for many years. Because their
time is so fully occupied and friends are reluctant to become

involved, social contacts may be drastically cut and the carer may virtually become a recluse. The boredom and monotony of a seemingly unending drudge can be debilitating both physically and emotionally.

Many carers are themselves elderly and in declining health, and the tasks of caring can cause further deterioration and general debilitation, or specific problems such as backache or injury caused by lifting the dependent person without assistance. Carers complain too that their physical appearance suffers, their hands and nails becoming rough and hard from washing. They may develop large arm muscles from lifting, or put on weight because they can no longer afford to eat such a well-balanced diet as they used to (Oliver 1984).

Both married and single people may find that their caring role puts severe limitations on sexual activity. Restrictions on time and money may mean that it is impossible to go out and meet new friends or socialise with existing contacts. Lack of privacy in the home and the demands of dependents may mean that opportunities for sexual activity are reduced or disappear entirely. Simple physical or emotional fatigue may dampen libido and impair sexual performance on occasions when an opportunity does arise. Just as people in general, professionals and others, seldom think about the sex lives of patients or assume that elderly or handicapped people have no sexual desires, so this aspect of carers' lives is often forgotten. Carers' sexual activity may be compromised because of the demands of the caring role but in addition, if the dependent is also the sexual partner, sexual relations may not be possible due to illness or treatment effects (see Chapters 6 and 7), and it is insensitive as well as useless for others to suggest having 'a cuddle instead' (Oliver 1984).

SEXUALITY AND CARING – THE OVERALL PICTURE

A reconsideration of the broad definition of sexuality which underlies our discussions makes it clear that informal caring is likely to have a profound impact on sexuality. Sexuality involves the total personality and is a part of how we see ourselves and others see us in all aspects of our lives. Self-concept and self-esteem are built up largely as we live out our social roles as workers, family members and gendered individuals. Our physical appearance and how we and others perceive this lead to the mental picture or body image we have of ourselves. As part of our personality, sexuality is closely related to sexual behaviour too. Positive body image and self-esteem both influence sexual desire and are reinforced by a satisfying sex life. The way we present ourselves and how others perceive us influence in turn who is attracted by us in a sexual sense. Sexual self-concept, libido, levels and kinds of sexual activity are also partly dependent on physical and mental health, and a sense of well-being in these areas will enhance sexual enjoyment. Conversely, poor body image and self-concept, a decline in physical or mental health, or lack of opportunity for sexual fulfilment will rebound on sex life, further reducing libido.

All of these negative changes can occur for carers in the community as direct results of the strains and deprivations involved in the caring role. Giving up or reducing outside employment means less money, fewer social contacts, and an endangered sense of independence and self-esteem. Standards of dress and grooming may suffer for financial reasons and lack of interest in the self, so that a negative body image results. Others may withdraw from carers both for fear of becoming involved in caring and in embarrassment at reduced circumstances. Former friends may resent that carers have less time for them, and be shocked at declining interest in personal presentation and social activities. Thus, contacts may be gradually lost and the resulting social isolation means that carers are thrown even more intensely into relationships with their dependents, and chances for social and sexual relationships outside of this disappear. Fatigue, both physical and emotional, may degenerate into frank depression, and loss of both libido and sexual outlets reinforce each other, with carers possibly ultimately seeing themselves and being seen by others as sexless and neutered (Oliver 1984). Finally, poor health and the changes of ageing may affect the sexuality of carers as well as their dependents.

The price of community care is a steep one to pay for many carers, whose sexual self-concept may be damaged very extensively and in a way that policy makers are either unaware of or decide to relegate to a subordinate position in the scale of costs.

BETTER COMMUNITY CARE

At the policy level, many changes can be envisaged which would help to make community care a truly higher quality form than routinised and impersonal institutional care. Supporting services could be available on a scale appropriate to need and on an equal

basis for all carers, women and men, single and married, employed and unemployed. The level and availability of social
security benefits would need to be greatly increased also, so that
people were not less well off financially when they chose to
become carers.

Community care of high quality may be the solution for many
carers and dependents, but not all relationships are such that they
can withstand the demands as well as build on the gains of
informal caring. Nor is it necessarily true that all institutions are
bad, and for some people independence may be greater in an
institution than in a home where they and carers are unhappy. An
elderly person living in a well-run and well-equipped block of
small flats supervised by a sympathetic warden, or in an informal
but comfortable residential hotel, may retain a good relationship
with a daughter with whom s/he would not get on if they were
obliged to live together. Imaginative experiments with a variety of
day care, short stay and residential facilities run by caring, flexible
and relaxed workers are needed to meet the different needs of a
society in which definitions of sexuality, sex roles and types of
'family' are changing.

Legislation to change social security benefits regulations could be
accompanied by new employment legislation to encourage em-
ployers to be more adaptable in granting time off for long or short
periods to carers, without loss of earnings, pension rights or
promotion opportunities. These arrangements should apply
equally to women and men, so that everyone wishing to combine
personal independence with a caring role could do so.

Without radical changes of this kind, community care will continue to be care 'on the cheap' (Opit 1978) which is paid for by
carers in a host of ways, including those affecting their sexuality.
Community care will also continue to treat women and men
differently if it remains based on unjustifiable assumptions about
appropriate sex role behaviour. Women and men will both remain
disadvantaged unless serious attention is given to ways of allow-
ing all humans to use their caring capacities and at the same time
retain their self-esteem.

CONCLUSION

Professional carers including, and perhaps especially, nurses have
an important role to play both in influencing community care
policies and in giving individualised care to clients in a way

which recognises the importance of sexuality in daily life. Our clients include informal carers because they receive professional nursing services, and the potential for nurses to develop their roles in this respect will grow enormously as social changes advance, the numbers of elderly people in the population increase, and more clients are nursed in the community.

Sexuality has not been a topic with which nurses or other health workers in this country have traditionally been concerned. In the last section of this book we shall look backwards to nursing history to see why this has happened, and look forward to see how nurses can fulfill their potential role in relation to sexuality in the future.

Nursing
&
Sexuality

CHAPTER 9

Sexuality and Nursing: The History of the Present

From early chronicles, through the Nightingale era, and right up to the present day, religious and domestic themes run through the history of nursing. To understand nursing today we need to look back at our history, not as a simple catalogue of events or as the achievements of a few pioneers or exceptional individuals, but as a process taking place within a wider society whose ideas and values have shaped what nursing has become. History is the study not of the simple unfolding of events but of social groups with their own schemes and purposes, working to ensure that their ideas are the ones which determine social developments. The history of the present can only be written by linking these social themes with nursing, rather than looking at nursing in isolation from the rest of society. In this chapter the theme of sexuality in nursing history will be traced, so that we can understand why even today's supposedly holistic models of care neglect this crucial aspect of health, while at the same time definitions of sexuality have a pervasive influence on nurses and nursing.

DEVOTION AND DOMESTICITY

Early nurses, both women and men, belonged to religious and secular orders of nuns and monks who had wards in their nunneries and monasteries where sick people were tended and shelter and rest were given to weary travellers. Tending the sick was part of a religious commitment to charitable work and caring for others in a setting of vocational dedication and self-denial (Bingham 1979), and the term 'sister' derives from these early religious links. But the majority of caring for the sick has always

127

taken place in people's own homes, as both trained and 'untrained' women cared for their own families and gave assistance and advice to neighbours.

Caring for women during pregnancy and attending childbirth were always seen as predominantly the realms of women, who may not have had formal training but who gained a wealth of experience and informal teaching from watching their own mothers and other women carrying out their work. Knowledge of herbal remedies and tried and tested treatments were passed down through the generations, when housekeeping was a highly-skilled and complex occupation involving not only cleaning and cooking but also skilled health care at a time when formal services were scarce and of dubious merit. Until the 18th century, medical 'science' was based on the teachings of Plato, Aristotle and Galen, and on Christian theology, and invoked ideas of humours and complexions, whereas care in the home given mainly by women was more truly scientific in its use of trials of remedies, observation of results, and learning from proven practitioners (Oakley 1976; Ehrehreich & English 1979; Versluysen 1980).

Industrialisation and urbanisation in the 18th and 19th centuries meant that large numbers of people who had previously grown their own food, made their living and organised their households on the fruits of their agricultural labour were dislocated from the land and flocked to the new and rapidly growing towns. Poverty forced many into workhouses where pauper nurses, both women and men, cared for their sick companions, again with little or no formal training and for minimal remuneration. Conditions in the workhouses were deliberately arranged to be a disincentive to the 'undeserving' poor, and pauper nurses sought to make the best of a bad job. The situation was therefore ripe for exploitation both of the nurses by the Poor Law Guardians, and of the sick by nurses. Hygienic conditions were very poor, food was unappetising and alcohol was administered on a rationing system. Nurses were thus able to improve their circumstances and make the most they could out of their position by charging other inmates for services and by stealing their food and taking their drink ration. Drinking was a widespread habit at the time, with ale served at mealtimes and a variety of drinks on sale in public houses. Therefore nurses were not unique in their drunkenness, as the Sara Gamp image portrayed by Dickens might suggest. Nevertheless, drunkenness in those who had charge of caring for sick people would have had particularly undesirable consequences, and it is not difficult to understand why nursing reformers placed such emphasis on sobriety and discipline.

THE AGE OF DISCIPLINE

The 19th century has been characterised as the age of discipline (Foucault 1977) because liberal reformers motivated by evangelical Christian ideas spearheaded reforms emphasising discipline in a wide range of areas from prisons to schools. Elizabeth Fry and many other Quakers were instrumental in organising regimes in prisons and mental hospitals based on the notion that 'gentling the masses' could be achieved not by force and physical punishment, but by discipline and inculcation of middle class standards of morality and behaviour. Thus, Elizabeth Fry's women prisoners were dressed in plain, serviceable dresses, wore no jewellery, and arranged their hair in severe styles covered by caps. Middle class women went into prisons to teach manners, domestic arts and childcare to incarcerated women, and religious teaching and church attendance were keystones of the regime. By following the role models provided by middle class Christian practitioners, prisoners were expected to turn from their rough ways and realise the benefits of soberness and an orderly way of life. Psychiatric patients in the newly-established 'Retreat' at York were treated in a similar manner which, while undoubtedly less physically severe than former methods, could be seen as harsh in that it sought to use the power hospital authorities had over patients to mould and discipline their personalities rather than their bodies. This is the interpretation made by Michel Foucault, a French scholar, who saw this use of power to control people through their 'souls' and way of life as the beginnings of a new kind of social control. He considers that this form of control is exercised widely today by 'intellectual police' in the form of psychiatrists, social workers, teachers, nurses and others, but above all by individuals everywhere exercising self-discipline because they know that 'the gaze' of the disciplinary power of the state is never far away.

Florence Nightingale's reform of nursing clearly fits easily into this scheme of things. Ladies were to be trained to take charge of hospitals and wards, and to supervise lower class nurses by strict discipline. When selecting potential nurses, morality and sobriety were fundamental criteria, and any breach of discipline or arguing with superiors meant instant dismissal. Florence Nightingale did not develop her ideas for a profession of nursing in a vacuum but in consort with the social thinking and reform movements in European society in general, and this no doubt allowed them to be accepted as the model for the organisation and training of the new profession.

FLORENCE NIGHTINGALE

Florence Nightingale's commitment to nursing was founded on a religious experience she underwent when she was frustrated by the inanities of existence as a lady in 'society' and was searching for a way to give meaning to her life. Her close friends were seriously committed High Church Anglicans and after receiving her 'call' she travelled with some of them in Europe, spending three months at Kaiserswerth in Germany, where a village pastor ran a training school for nurse-deaconesses which was marked by its high moral tone and devotion to duty. Elizabeth Fry had visited Kaiserswerth earlier and had been impressed enough to incorporate in her own methods the idea of training peasant women through a life of simple frugality (Bingham 1977).

The qualities considered necessary for nurses at that time included a 'holy' nature, self-effacement, soberness, chastity, charitableness and guilelessness (Gamarnikov 1978), which were the stereotypes of a middle-class woman of the Victorian era, and Nightingale's statement that to be a good nurse one must be a good woman expresses this link between femininity and nursing, as well as emphasising character as the most important element in a nurse. She also likened nursing to motherhood, stating that sick adults were very much like children in need of care. Like Elizabeth Fry's prisoners, Florence Nightingale's nurses were plainly dressed, wore no flowers or decorations, and were strictly chaperoned on duty by their ward sister and off duty by a housekeeper.

The fact that Nightingale's first nurses worked in a military setting added further disciplinary influences to her thinking for two main reasons. Firstly, the new nurses were to travel abroad as a group of women living and working amongst men soldiers, from whose uncouth ways they were deemed to need protection. Secondly, acceptance of the nurses by the army was hard-won and Florence Nightingale wanted to be sure that their position would not be prejudiced by encroaching on the army doctors' sphere of responsibility. If doctors thought nurses were taking over their role, exercising initiative and taking independent decisions, the whole mission would be thwarted and the nurses would be sent back to

England. Not only would much needed care not be given to the thousand of injured and dying soldiers, but the very status and development of the new profession for women would be put in jeopardy. The nurse was therefore to be the 'handmaiden' of the doctor, a term which means literally a maiden who is a 'hand', or in other words a female domestic servant (Austin 1977).

The work done by the nurses was therefore strictly demarcated by Florence Nightingale to exclude 'medical' tasks and to focus on 'the sanitary idea'. She stated that the function of nurses was to put patients in the best position for nature's healing work to progress unhampered, and therefore 'nursing of the room', cleanliness and ventilation, together with hygiene and nutrition of the patients, were paramount (Gamarnikov 1978; Bingham 1979). Once again, then, the definitions of women and nurses, and their 'proper' attributes and work, coincided in a way that was rarely challenged until the Salmon Report (HMSO 1966) removed domestic work from the control of nurses.

A WOMAN OF HER TIME

Florence Nightingale was truly a woman of her age and although she was an exceptional woman in some ways, in others she conformed to Victorian stereotypes of femininity (Austin 1977). Her father had educated her and her sister Parthenhope, which led Florence to be deeply dissatisfied with the superficial pleasures of life as a beautiful 'society' lady rich enough to live comfortably and idly in a large country house and to go to London for 'the season'. Her rejection of marriage and pursuit of a career – then a rare course for a rich woman – has led to speculation that she was a lesbian, but it seems more plausible to see her as the archetype of a Victorian lady who, whilst achieving more than most others in her search for a meaningful role in life, was unable to throw off the chains of oppressive cultural mores.

Idleness for middle class women was an invention of Victorian industrial society. A man's success in business and the amount of wealth he built up was testified by the degree of luxury in which he and his family lived. Conspicuous consumption in the form of a big house, carriages, servants, and above all a beautiful and lavishly-dressed wife to adorn the home and provide children, were the distinguishing marks of success and status. This life-style, however, was a dubious privilege for women, who passed their time playing music, sewing and entertaining, but had little worthwhile activity to give a sense of meaning and fulfilment to their lives (Stark 1979). The burden of repeated childbirth added to their physical and emotional weariness and many middle class women went into a 'decline', taking to their beds while their working class sisters worked long hours for pitiful wages in dirty, noisy and dangerous factories (Ehrenreich & English 1979).

Elizabeth Barrett Browning, the writer, and Harriet Martineau, the politicial economist, were two other educated, middle class women who took to their beds as did Florence Nightingale from 1859 to her death in 1910. It seems clear that she had no physical complaint, although she herself was afraid she had a heart condition because she experienced chest pain, palpitations and difficulty in breathing at the very thought of entertaining family visitors. Invalidity was a refuge for women who could not tolerate the reality of their lives in Victorian middle class society. For some, the sheer weight of boredom, or the exhaustion caused by submitting to their husbands' sexual demands and the inevitable string of pregnancies which resulted, provoked a reaction so great that they withdrew into the isolation of their bedrooms as a way of gaining some control over their own lives. An obvious parallel could be drawn with today's depressed housewife, who may use alcohol as a means of escape from the routine of housework and lack of stimulating work or company.

Florence Nightingale may have been depressed when she returned to England from the Crimea, both because she was physically exhausted and had been under a great deal of stress in her work, but also perhaps because of the very different prospects which lay ahead of her in returning to 'society' and its trivial round of engagements after an experience such as she had had. As time passed, however, Nightingale used her 'illness' to manipulate politicians, doctors and nurses to come and visit her, listen to her views, and adopt her ideas for sanitary reform, establishing nursing schools, and campaigning against registration of nurses. Although confined to bed or a chair, she invested immense intellectual and physical energy in her political work and writing, and it is hard to accept her own view of herself as a weak and sick woman. A more plausible interpretation might be that, restricted by Victorian expectations of how 'true femininity' should be expressed, she exploited these very stereotypes of grace, fragility and emotionality in order to crush those who disagreed with her but were too refined to oppose an invalid lady. It has been suggested that she adopted this strategy in a completely conscious way and took a morbid pleasure in her own weakness (Cannedy 1979). If this interpretation is accepted, Florence Nightingale was indeed the 'ideal' woman of her age for, although she was unconventional in demanding an independent career, she nevertheless conformed to and promoted conventional stereotypes of femininity both in her own behaviour and in selecting and training nurses, and in organising the fledgeling profession of nursing (Gamarnikov 1978).

The themes of vocation, obedience and the nurse as woman, wife and mother whose natural role of carer and domestic worker ideally suited her for nursing, continued to run through nursing history in this century. They were very much in evidence in the struggle for registration, with both sides in the debate agreeing that the nursing role should be subservient to the medical one. But the anti-registrationists, of whom Florence Nightingale was one, feared that registered nurses would come to see themselves as professional colleagues of doctors and not the executors of medical orders. Thus from religious beginnings, with monks performing the 'laying on of hands' on the sick assisted by nuns, to the mid-1960s nursing was defined as women's work to be administered by women. Men played a role in nursing from the start, and were used as attendants in Poor Law asylums and later in psychiatric hospitals, principally because their superior physical strength equipped them to control unruly patients. However, a separate Register for male nurses was kept and the Royal College of Nursing only admitted men as members in 1960 (Austin 1977). Men remained the minority in nursing even in psychiatric hospitals and, in posts of responsibility from the ward sister or charge nurse level upwards, nursing was overwhelmingly a female profession and its subordinate status to the male-dominated medical profession was thereby guaranteed.

SALMONISATION = MASCULINISATION

By the 1960s the problem of high drop-out rates during nurse training was causing continued anxiety both within and outside the profession. Debates continued over whether the shortage of nurses was in fact due to a failure to recruit sufficient entrants, whether the real problem lay in the well-documented rigid discipline, hierarchical and impersonal relationships both between nurses and patients, and among nurses, or whether 'non-nursing duties' were to blame. Menzies (1970) had shown that authoritarian treatment of nurses, who bore a heavy burden of responsibility on duty but were subject to petty regulations in nurses' homes, caused much stress, and the introduction of the assistant nurse grade had done little to ensure that nurses spent their time on 'real nursing' rather than routine cleaning jobs. Furthermore, those who devoted themselves to a lifelong career in nursing could see no clear and rewarding career structure laid out before them (HMSO 1966).

Therefore the government set up a committee with Brian Salmon in the chair, briefed to look into Senior Nursing Staff Structure. Salmon had had a career in industry, another member, TT Paterson, was a professor of business management, and the only other non-nurse member was a medical administrator. Thus, although nurses were a majority on the committee, it appears that the government had already decided the outcome by choosing these three members, and that its intention was to introduce into nursing a managerial model which had already been put into operation in local government and education (Cockburn 1977; Webb 1981).

The Salmon Report, published in 1966, was severely critical of the style of female, generalist administration which had characterized nursing up to that point. Women nurse administrators were said to be unable to delegate or to take decisions, and to be over-concerned with trivial details. Mick Carpenter (1977), a nurse and historian, calls the Salmon Report openly sexist in posing its criticism of female nurses in this way, and in advocating a style of 'scientific management' more suited to men, who "find it easier to stand the physical and nervous strain of the top jobs than many women do" (HMSO 1966). Nurses on the Salmon Committee accepted the proposals because they seemed to offer the promise of enhanced professional status for nurses in relation to doctors, and greater influence in hospital management. Domestic duties were taken out of nurses' jurisdiction and put in the charge of administrators, and a clear, hierarchical promotion structure was drawn up.

The trend which was initiated in 1966 found further expression in the 1974 and subsequent reorganisations of the health service, with their advocacy of management theory and introduction of industrial-type philosophies. These changes have led to a complete turn-round in nursing so that, whereas previously nursing was subordinate to the male medical profession and controlled from within by the upper-class successors of Nightingale's lady nurses, from Salmon onwards it has become entirely male-dominated (Austin 1977; Carpenter 1977). Medical superordination continues but male nurse managers are increasingly appointed so that, by 1982, 43.8 per cent of District Nursing Officer posts and 50.5 per cent of Director of Nurse Education positions were held by men (Nuttall 1983). In psychiatric hospitals men constituted 41.9 per cent of nurse administrators in 1959 but 79.8 per cent in 1979 (Pollock & West 1984). Men make up approximately 10 per cent of all entrants to general nursing and 32 per cent of entrants to psychiatric nursing, but they now predominate in all top management posts.

Mick Carpenter and others see this 'male takeover' (Nuttall 1983) as detrimental to both nursing and its clients. Managerial values are those of rationality and 'objective' decision-making uninfluenced by emotion, and men are better placed to apply for management posts because their socialisation along the lines of cultural stereotypes of masculinity makes it likely that they will possess these characteristics to a greater degree than women. They also stay longer in nursing without a break, work full-time more often than women, and have greater geographical mobility (Carpenter 1977). Women, on the other hand, have learned that they are expected to be more attracted and suited to bedside nursing and 'housekeeping' tasks, to give up full-time work to raise their families, and to move according to the requirements of their husbands' jobs (Austin 1977; Nuttall 1983; Pollock & West 1984). So women nurses are less likely to see themselves as suited to managerial jobs and to be less qualified because of shorter previous service.

Whether patients and clients benefit from the encroachment of 'masculine' ways of thinking and behaving in nursing is doubted by most writers who accept this underlying explanation of recent nursing history. Caring requires attributes of gentleness, the ability to feel emotional reactions in order to be able to put oneself in the place of a sufferer and make a constructive contribution to easing pain and discomfort, and a capacity to put others first and remain patient even when one is exhausted by physical and emotional strain. But these abilities are not sufficient unless they are accompanied by knowledge of the processes of human behaviour and body functions in health and disease. Neither of these kinds of attributes are inherently the province of either women or men, and both are potentially equally able to be caring and intelligent nurses. Only when the stereotypes come into play, teaching people how they 'ought' to behave and do their jobs, do things go wrong in the way they seem to have done since managerial ideologies came to the bedside, as Mick Carpenter (1977) and Rita Austin (1977) suggest. Summarising this view, Robert Dingwall (1979) states

> "The enhanced masculinity of nursing benefits neither the patients who have to suffer it, nor the staff who have to work it, nor the society in which it is located".

IMAGES OF NURSING TODAY

Images of nurses from the past force themselves upon us still today, as a visit to a paperback bookshop soon confirms. Either the innocent, dedicated and sexually-inexperienced nurse at last succumbs to the passionate embraces of Dr X, or the happy-go-lucky, randy nurse, whose short skirt reveals her black suspenders, is the life and soul of the medical residence. Television soap operas and films shown in cinemas in decaying parts of town portray the same stereotypes, which are easily recognisable as the madonna/whore paradox of Christian religion (Muff 1982) or the pre- and post-Nightingale caricatures of nurses as drunken and loose-living sluts or pure and dedicated women single-mindedly pursuing their vocation.

Above all, images of nurses are images of women, whether flattering or not. The man who is a nurse is still an object of surprise if not derision, as the very term 'male nurse' implies. If a man is a nurse, doing 'women's work, then his status as a 'real' man is in question, but his manhood can be restored by giving him the title *male* nurse. The same happens with women doctors, who are still considered unusual enough for the special term 'lady doctor' to be used to refer to them. Research has shown, however, that people judge women who go into medicine as less socially deviant than men who become nurses (Hesselbart 1977), probably because anyone who chooses a low-status occupation when he has the possibility of doing better for himself is considered to be particularly strange. Many men in nursing are deeply hurt by this stereotyping and by frequent innuendos about their sexuality, which imply that they are homosexual and therefore perverted or deviant. Such attitudes are based on inaccurate understanding and prejudice both about nursing and the personal qualities which make people good nurses, and about homosexual people (see Chapter 1).

Concepts of appropriate work for female and male nurses mirror definitions of sex-roles in wider society. Women nursing students may be allocated to a gynaecology ward while men go to genito-urinary wards or sexually transmitted diseases clinics, and until the Sex Discrimination Act 1975 men were not allowed to train as midwives. Male-midwife, incidentally, is a term with a long history and was originally used to distinguish untrained male accoucheurs from medical practitioners whose main methods consisted of interventions in labour with instruments (Oakley 1976). 'Midwife' means literally 'with woman' and so can apply to any person who helps a woman in labour. In psychiatric nursing, women tend to focus attention more on keeping busy with housework-type tasks while men get on with the office work and deal with finances, off-duty and administrative procedures (Pollock & West 1984). Few men enter paediatric nursing, in the same way that they avoid nursery and primary school teaching because childcare is a woman's sphere par excellence (Deem 1978), and the home-centred activities of district nursing and health visiting are overwhelmingly done by women nurses. We have also seen earlier in this chapter that higher levels of management and nurse education attract considerably more men than would be representative of their numbers in the profession as a whole.

The most visible intrusion of gender stereotypes into everyday nursing life comes in the form of nurses' uniforms. Women wear dresses, often with tight belts but always revealing their legs, which are culturally defined as sexually provocative even when not in black stockings. Most female nurses still wear decorative and entirely non-functional caps designed to enhance their 'femininity' and attractiveness, but like Florence Nightingale's recruits they must not use jewellery or 'excessive' make-up and should strive for a demure appearance. Men, on the other hand, wear comfortable and functional trousers, loose-fitting smock-tops and no frilly cap so that, unlike their female colleagues, they can lift patients and bend down without having their movements dangerously impaired by restrictive clothing and without revealing parts of the body normally kept covered in everyday social life. Traditional, ornate nurses' uniforms for women turn them into sexual objects in exactly the same way as contestants in 'beauty' contests are displayed in a manner calculated to be sexually provocative, and we see again the paradox of the nurse and woman as simultaneously innocent and titillating.

PLAYING AT NURSES AND DOCTORS

The doctor-nurse game was first described in print in 1976 (Stein 1976) but was familiar to nurses long before that. In the 'game', the doctor takes decisions and is in charge, but he needs the nurse to give him information on which to base his decisions and to carry out his orders. To keep up the appearance of being in control but not get into difficulties, the wise doctor listens to 'his' nurses and weighs up what they have to say, and in return the 'good' nurse does not reveal how much she knows and how much power she could exercise if she chose. So she plays the game by hinting and suggesting tentatively what the patient's problem might be, using her 'feminine wiles' in true Nightingale fashion. The doctor reciprocates by assuming responsibility and appearing to take decisions, all the while using the nurse as a tool for carrying out his job. For example, a nurse may notice that a patient taking an antibiotic has developed a skin reaction and she may consider that a change of drug and a prescription for an anti-histamine cream would be appropriate. However, she would not dream of coming right out and saying this to the doctor, so when he reaches the patient on the ward round, she might say, 'Oh dear, Mr Smith, you do look blotchy. Try not to scratch, dear. What could be the matter, doctor? I wonder if it's something he's allergic to?' The doctor will probably then say something like 'Perhaps it's a reaction to a drug. Pass me his prescription sheet, nurse. Oh yes, I expect it's this antibiotic. We'll change that for you, Mr Smith, and nurse will give you some cream to stop the itching.' Thus, when all participants play the game according to the rules, life in the ward runs smoothly and nobody looses points. On the other hand, if a player breaks the rules and speaks out of turn, the game is disrupted and somebody wins at the expense of the other player. The player who has lost will then be on the look-out for an opportunity to win back the advantage and the social atmosphere of the ward will be strained.

Doctor-nurse relations and the division of labour between them remain largely as Florence Nightingale agreed with doctors that they should be. Nurses are still subject to doctors' control and it is not only patients who are 'under doctors' orders'. Nurses, like wives, prepare both trolleys for procedures and trays of coffee for doctors, help them to carry out their work quickly and with as little effort as possible by filling in forms, taking specimens for them, and smoothing their paths in patient encounters, just as a wife or housekeeper performs services for her husband or employer. After the doctor has moved on, the nurse clears up after him, both by cleaning and disposing of equipment and by talking to patients to explain what the doctor may have said too quickly or in language too technical to understand, and by filling information gaps left as the doctor hurried on to his next patient (Webb 1984b).

The doctor–nurse–patient triad transports the man–wife–child group from the home to the health care setting (Gamarnikov 1978; Muff 1982). The male–father–doctor initiates action and controls the other participants, the wife–mother–nurse provides him with material services and emotional support in return for a relatively secure job, and the child–patient has the lowest status, being expected to remain passive, do as doctor daddy says, and be well-behaved. Following cultural stereotypes of sex-role behaviour, male doctors exercise scientific methods to cure patients while female nurses use their softer, feminine and maternal 'natures' to care for the sick, and male nurses and female doctors are embarrassing complications which disturb the smooth surface of social expectations.

Sexuality is therefore an important factor in nursing and health care. As with all stereotypes, those which operate in this context are wasteful of women's and men's caring and intellectual capacities and hurtful to their self-concepts. Self-expression is curbed and prejudice given free-rein when men are openly or covertly discouraged from tackling the kinds of nursing work they could do well and from which they would gain immense satisfaction (Brookfield et al 1982). The same problems confront men who want to share more equally in caring for their own and other people's children at home or in paid employment. At the same time, women often fail to achieve their potential because they have learned that it is not feminine to be ambitious, or because their family-centred life-style cuts them off from advancement at work. Doctors and nurses do not work in teams of equals, each giving the other's opinions the hearing and respect they deserve and facilitating open discussion, because sexist stereotypes intervene in their relationships.

History has led us to a position in which sexuality plays a determining role in health care but, simultaneously, fundamental issues of sexuality are neglected for professionals and patients alike. Holistic care is much discussed but little practised, at least in respect of sexuality, as research with doctors and nurses has shown.

RESEARCH ON SEXUALITY AND NURSING

The more knowledge people have about human sexuality, the more open and flexible they are likely to be in their attitudes towards their own and others' behaviour, and their personal development and interpersonal relationships will benefit as well as their professional work. For health professionals this increased knowledge, and the greater security in one's own sexuality it brings, allows them to be more at ease in professional situations with sexual implications (Lief & Payne 1975). An American nurse studying the knowledge and attitudes of students towards sexuality using a Sexual Knowledge and Attitudes Test (SKAT) found that both female nursing students and qualified nurses were less knowledgeable and more conservative than female medical students (Payne 1976). Registered nurses were the most conservative of all and family planning nurses scored lower than nursing students. Family planning nurses were included in the study because they might be expected to be more knowledgeable and open about sexuality since their work is so closely involved with this topic. Age and social class influenced results on the SKAT, so that younger nurses and those from higher social classes had more knowledge and more liberal attitudes, but religion did not appear to be influential, Roman Catholics not being scored as more conservative as might be expected. However, regular church attenders and those coming from non-urban areas were less knowledgeable and more conservative in their attitudes.

In another study in the USA, Kuczynski (1980) also used the SKAT and again found that registered nurses were more conservative than second year medical students, although their comparative knowledge levels were the same. As medical students progressed in their training, registered nurses would be likely to fall behind in knowledge as in Payne's study. Kuczynski also found that the nurses had less knowledge and less liberal attitudes towards sexuality than non-medical post-graduate students.

Both these studies confirm the report of a World Health Organisation seminar on 'The Teaching of Human Sexuality in Schools for Health Professionals', which states:

> "Of all forms of health education, the provision of advice and instruction in matters relating to sexual behaviour demands the greatest tact, integrity, tolerance and understanding of human behaviour and personal relationships. Members of the health professions, although frequently asked for help by people with difficul-

ties in their sex lives, are often ill-equipped with the knowledge and
skills needed for counselling in human sexuality, sexual behaviour,
family planning, etc., and may be reticent about giving such advice
or unwilling to do so."
(Mace *et al* 1974)

The great areas of ignorance about sexuality found in these two
American studies suggest that teaching on this topic needs to be
included in nursing education, which often does not go beyond
the biological aspects of reproduction (Lief & Payne 1975). But
knowledge alone does not necessarily lead to attitude change, and
an underlying philosophy that accepts sexuality as important in
health care is needed so that the subject is integrated into all stages
of teaching and giving nursing care (Kuczynski 1980). In this way,
and through the use of experiential teaching methods, films and
group discussions, an atmosphere of acceptance can be promoted
which will encourage students to examine their own values and
gain the security and self-acceptance which can allow them to be
comfortable in dealing with sexuality in patient care (Payne 1976).

No studies like these of nurses' knowledge and attitudes towards
sexuality in health care have been done in the UK, but other
research suggests that findings would be similar. For example,
district nurses in 1980 were reported to spend only 17 per cent of
their time with patients on giving advice, counselling, reassurance
and education, compared with 40 per cent of time spent on
technical procedures and 38 per cent on other nursing care. When
asked which areas of counselling and health education they would
like to spend more time on, only 2 per cent of the district nurses
mentioned marital and psychosexual counselling, while 41 per
cent did not name any area on which they would like to spend
more time in this way (Dunnell *et al* 1982). As a prominent writer
on sexuality in medical education points out, saying nothing is
also a form of counselling because silence conveys the message
that the topic is not important enough to merit discussion (Lief
1970).

Other research in this country also tends to confirm the American
findings. Women having gynaecological surgery are particularly in
need of information and advice about the implications of their
operations for sexuality. They have heard 'old wives' tales' and
prophecies of doom which make them wonder if a hysterectomy,
for example, will cause them to grow hair on their faces, put on
weight, become unattractive to their sexual partners, and lose all
their own sexual urges and feelings of pleasure. They also worry

at somehow they will feel less of a woman', 'empty inside', or 'just like a shell' (Webb 1983). They desperately need accurate information to put their minds at rest and to help them manage their surgery and recovery in ways which disrupt other aspects of sexuality as little as possible, including their home-centred roles as wives and mothers, their work outside the home, and their social life (Webb 1984a). When in hospital for a hysterectomy, however, women are often disappointed and critical about the lack of help of this kind given by nurses and doctors. Instead of the detailed information and advice they want about what the operation entails, what effects to expect, and how to build up activities again afterwards, they are given only brief hints about 'no lifting', 'don't do too much', and 'take it easy'. These items merely tell them what *not* to do, so that they are left in the dark about what they *should* do, and resuming sexual activity after the operation is often neglected in the same way (Webb 1983).

Nurses working in specialities where sexuality is an important issue would be expected to realise that their patients have these concerns, and to have the necessary knowledge, skills and attitudes to respond to their needs. A study of trained nurses working on gynaecology wards in one city in England confirmed that nurses did define sexuality and giving support and counselling to patients as vital, if not the most essential, features of work in this speciality (Webb 1985c). They had talked to their patients and were aware that they feared 'losing their womanhood', but nurses interpreted this as referring only to patients' sex lives and not to wider aspects of sexuality, self-concept and self-esteem. When asked what advice and information they would give to a woman going home from hospital after a hysterectomy, these nurses confirmed what patients had said in an earlier study (Webb 1983) about small pieces of prohibitive information on general activities, and they rarely mentioned advice on resuming sex life. Not one of the 30 nurses interviewed mentioned general issues of sexuality or emotional factors as needing discussion when preparing patients for discharge.

Gynaecological nurses in this study had very ambivalent attitudes towards their patients as women (Webb 1984b). On the one hand they felt that, as women themselves, they were uniquely placed to understand how their patients felt, because 'After all, you're a woman yourself and you've gone through some of these things – PMT, period pains, etc.'. On the other hand they expressed denigrating and unsympathetic responses. They felt that gynaecology patients tended to 'make the most of it' to 'think they're only here for a rest and we're supposed to wait on them', and to exploit the emotional aspects of their problems to gain attention from their husbands and ward staff. The strongest attitudes of condemnation were reserved for abortion patients, who were seen as manipulative and lying in order to secure an abortion 'just because it's inconvenient' to have a fourth child or to be pregnant at the age of 15. Abortion patients were considered simply not to bother with contraception, but to come for repeated terminations of pregnancy as a method of birth control and to feel no guilt or regret. Rather, they were 'brazen' and 'little madams' who boasted about their situation.

Research with women undergoing termination of pregnancy (TOP) contradicts these interpretations. Repeat abortions are relatively few, and it is rare for women to treat TOP lightly. More commonly, having the abortion is a lonely and painful business because women are ashamed and embarrassed to tell their family and friends of their predicament, and therefore have nobody to help them work through their conflicts (Webb 1985a). Arranging an abortion can be very difficult and late terminations, which were of course especially distasteful to nurses, may result from delays in being referred to a specialist or other administrative hold-ups. Perhaps it is not surprising that in their desperation women become very emotionally upset and appear demanding and un-reasonable to hospital staff.

Looking at the situation from the point of view of gynaecological nurses, their feelings and reactions also seem to be reasonable responses to the position in which they find themselves. The majority of nurses in the study had not chosen to work on gynaecology wards, but had gone there because that was the only post available when they were looking for a new job. In relation to abortion patients, they had very little control over their work and consequently gained little satisfaction from it. Often patients' notes were incomplete and gave no basis for understanding how the decision to do a TOP was taken. Therefore nurses could not emphathise with the problems faced, for example, by a young woman with three children, whose husband was unemployed and drank excessively, when she found herself pregnant again and felt she could not cope with another child on top of her existing burdens. TOP patients stayed in hospital for a very short time, which increased nursing workload, and nurses had no role in abortion and contraception counselling. Therefore the nurses felt they were being used to carry out other people's decisions, and that they had little influence on decision-making and little role to play with these patients beyond preparing them for operation and looking after them in the early recovery phase.

Although nurses working in this special field wanted to play a counselling and educative role, they had not been trained to do so. Only three of the thirty interviewed in this study had had any preparation in communications skills, and for two of these the session had lasted one hour. The third nurse was a Registered Mental Nurse who had had this training as part of her psychiatric experience. Special preparation for work on gynaecology wards had consisted of learning anatomy and physiology, and a few hours of lectures during basic training by doctors and nurse teachers about gynaecological conditions and treatments. Post-basic training specifically to prepare them for their work on gynaecology wards had not been given.

CONCLUSION

In the light of these studies, which grow out of a nursing history fraught with sexual repression and stereotyping (Hogan 1980), it is hardly surprising that nurses do not have high knowledge levels and open attitudes towards sexuality in health care, nor the necessary skills which would allow them to give information and counselling to patients. It is therefore unjust to criticise the care they give when their professional education has not equipped them to carry out their work in ways which respond to patients' needs and which allow them to enhance their own self-esteem and job satisfaction. Nor is it hard to understand their lack of enthusiasm when they have no choice over their area of work, no influence in what happens to patients, and little background knowledge of how decision-making is done.

To remedy this, all nurses need an educational background which gives them knowledge of the biological and psychological aspects of sexual development, the reproductive process, varieties of sexual expression, sexual dysfunctions and cultural aspects of sex, marriage and the family (Mace *et al* 1974). As well as knowledge, questions of values need to be studied, because nurses cannot be effective if they do not develop an understanding of the moral, aesthetic and religious sensibilities of the people with whom they will deal, and with their own values and beliefs (Payne 1976). Skills are also needed in assessing, intervening, teaching and counselling individuals and groups (Hogan 1980), and experiential learning rather than formal teaching methods provide the most favourable way to approach these topics in a nursing curriculum (Hogan 1980, Weinberg 1982).

Janie Weinberg wrote a textbook on sexuality in nursing practice because she believed that:

> "Nursing is in a unique position to provide for the sexual health care needs of patients. This care is appropriate to the goals of health promotion and primary prevention in nursing. It allows nurses to function as advocates for clients, and enables them to meet the growing demand for informed, responsible patient care."
> (Weinberg 1982)

If nurses learned about the biological, psychological and sociological aspects of sexuality and its influence in our daily lives, patient care would undoubtedly improve and nurses would achieve a greater sense of fulfillment from their work. Professional relationships within nursing, and between nurses and doctors, which are the product of a long history of prejudice and manipulation on both sides, could be better understood and efforts could be made to change oppressive attitudes and behaviour at work, building on greater knowledge and on training in communications skills including assertiveness training (Henley & Freeman 1982; Smythe 1982). The enhanced personal and professional self-esteem nurses would gain from greater awareness, openness and autonomy would in turn feed back into the quality of nursing care.

These are enormous and challenging issues and one book can only begin to open them up for discussion. So far the emphasis has been on the 'knowledge' aspects of sexuality in society in general, and in nursing and health care in particular. In the final chapters, we shall turn to the role of nurses in planning and giving care which acknowledges and respects the sexuality of patients and nurses alike.

CHAPTER 10

Sexuality in Nursing Care

Sexuality involves the totality of being a person and therefore nurses and patients are only given their full respect as people when nursing care has firm foundations in a truly holistic approach incorporating sexuality as a vital aspect of humanity. If the definition of sexuality underlying this book is accepted, then it becomes essential for all nurses to integrate the concept of sexuality into their nursing care. Throughout all stages of the process of assessing, planning, giving and evaluating care, we need to be alert to cues which draw attention to people's problems in relation to sexuality and to use nursing judgement about the kinds of help needed. For the majority of patients or clients, the greatest needs are to express their feelings, to have their concerns acknowledged as valid, and to be given the information they need to manage their lives. All nurses have a role to play at this level of care, and to be able to fulfill this role confidently and competently they need to be knowledgeable about the biological, psychological and social aspects of sexuality which have been the focus of earlier chapters.

In this chapter, we shall discuss the attitudes and skills which complement sound knowledge and allow nurses to give care effectively and to feel secure in their personal and professional judgements. The application of these skills will be traced through the stages of the nursing process.

SEXUALITY AND THE NURSE

As members of a society with widely accepted myths and stereotypes about sexuality, nurses have the same queries, doubts

147

and emotions as their patients and clients, and their own personal moral values. A basic nursing ethic, however, is that of professional neutrality, which means that all clients should be treated alike, and that neither the client's nor nurse's personal beliefs should influence the care that is given (UKCC 1983). This means that heterosexual and homosexual clients, victims of violence and their assailants, women wanting to conceive and those wanting an abortion have the right to receive high quality care irrespective of their personal background and beliefs.

Being non-judgemental does not mean giving up personal beliefs or changing them to fit in with what other people think is morally right (Goldsborough 1970). Very much to the contrary, it means becoming aware of personal values, taking them out and examining them, and deciding how important they are. To do this we need to be aware of alternative moral positions and to compare these with our own beliefs, weighing up the positive and negative aspects of different philosophies of life and making informed decisions about which principles to use in making personal decisions. Discussing moral questions with others, challenging their beliefs and defending our own are powerful ways to reach self-understanding and self-acceptance, but this is only possible if debates are held in an open and accepting atmosphere, where nobody is judged or ridiculed for their views, and everyone feels safe in testing out their beliefs.

In schools of nursing, moral issues are often discussed in this way as part of the process of learning to be a nurse. Euthanasia, abortion, resuscitation of deformed babies and maintenance of unconscious patients on life-support systems are examples of topics which feature in nurse education programmes. Sexuality is an issue which urgently needs to be included in these debates too, for it affects us all as people and as care-givers, and its neglect can cause a great deal of stress and distress for nurses, as it did for the gynaecology nurses in the study described in Chapter 9 (Webb 1985c).

'Values clarification' exercises can be used to initiate group discussions about moral questions, but can be productive when done by individuals too. These exercises involve answering a number of questions and paying attention not only to the answers but also to the personal thoughts and emotions they bring up. There are no right or wrong answers to the questions, which are designed to develop self-awareness of feelings that influence behaviour and which may previously have gone unacknowledged. The rationale behind the exercises is that, by becoming aware of attitudes and their influence on our behaviour, people can monitor their responses in real-life situations. For nurses working with patients and clients whose values and life-styles often differ greatly from their own, this suspension of judgemental reactions is a professional necessity, and practice in achieving it can help self-control in challenging situations. Some examples of values clarification questions about sexuality are illustrated in Figure 10.1.

How do you feel about discussing sexual topics in mixed company?
How do you feel about discussing sexual topics in front of children?
How do you feel when you hear dirty or obscene jokes?
How do you feel when you hear people using sexual terms when they are swearing?
What feelings do the following words bring up for you:
Penis   vagina   masturbation   homosexual
How would you feel if a male patient touched you while you were washing him?
How would you feel if a female patient touched you while you were washing her?
Have you ever examined your own genitalia with a mirror?
If you did this, would you feel embarrassed, ashamed, perverted, childish, pleased, proud, sexually excited?
How do you feel when you see children playing on the beach with no clothes on?
How do you feel when you see pictures of naked people?
How do you feel when you see explicit sexual acts in films or on television?

Figure 10.1 Values clarification exercise

Nurses who are knowledgeable and have learned to accept their own and other people's feelings and beliefs about sexuality will be more comfortable in dealing both with professional situations having sexual connotations, such as washing patients of the opposite sex, and with broader issues of sexuality like working with abortion patients or in contraception clinics. Becoming secure in one's beliefs is an essential prerequisite to taking morally-based decisions in professional life and asserting one's right not to participate in acts which go against one's personal values. The 'conscientious objection' clause in abortion legislation is rarely invoked, for example, although many nurses are not happy to work with these patients (Webb 1985c). If, through wider discussion of moral questions in nurse education, more nurses felt able to make their objections known and to exert their right not to work in certain settings, nurses would grow in personal and professional stature. At the same time, standards of nursing care would be enhanced because those working in sensitive areas would be there because they had made an informed decision that this kind of work was right for them. Their positive attitudes would influence the care they gave in the same way as negative attitudes influence what happens to 'unpopular' patients (Stockwell 1972; Kelly & May 1982).

Nobody is unbiassed about sexuality or any other topic which raises moral questions, and nurses are no exception. Many nurses have entered the profession precisely because they hold strong beliefs about the value of human life and the prevention of suffering. Sexuality is just one area among many others in which knowledge and self-awareness will foster respect for patients' rights and needs. Giving high quality, non-judgemental care will also help to build nurses' self-esteem as individuals and as professionals (Goldsborough 1970; Smythe 1982; Bush & Kjervik 1979).

TAKING A NURSING HISTORY

Questions about sexuality are needed when taking a nursing history from patients and clients because sexuality is part of the total personality, and influences thoughts and behaviour in health, illness and disability. The section of the nursing assessment relating to sexuality will be relatively brief in the majority of instances, its aim being to pick up cues about the interplay between sexuality, health and illness in a particular individual. A detailed history of sexual development and practices from childhood to the present is not required unless a client has a particular sexual problem which has been brought to light by a request for treatment or has emerged in the course of a medical examination or nursing assessment. In a case like this, the client will be referred to an appropriate therapist who is trained and skilled in this speciality and who may also have a basic training in nursing, medicine, psychiatry or psychology. (For an example of a detailed, specialist assessment of sexuality *see* Weinberg 1982, 29–33.)

Questions used in a nursing assessment should follow a pattern starting with general topics and gradually focussing in more detail on particular aspects of sexuality and sexual behaviour. In this way, rapport is built up as straightforward questions are raised, and the patient or client and the nurse feel at ease when those of a more personal and intimate nature are reached. Questions should be clearly related to the person's health or illness problems, so that their relevance is obvious and there is no suggestion that intrusive information is being sought unnecessarily. These guidelines, of course, apply equally to any part of a nursing history and a nurse should always be ready to omit questions judged inappropriate to a particular patient or client, or to explain why the question is being asked. Guidelines for taking a nursing history are given in Figure 10.2, but the kinds of questions and their position in the overall assessment will depend on the conceptual framework used as a basis for nursing care. Some assessment frameworks, for example that of Roper, Logan and Tierney (1983), include a separate section on sexuality, but with others questions about sexuality need to be inserted at appropriate points in the assessment, as in the case of Roy's Adaptation Model (Riehl & Roy 1980) or the Orem Self-Care Model (Orem 1980). Example care plans using two of these models are included later in this chapter.

The method of taking a nursing history which includes questions about sexuality is similar to that for every nursing history. Privacy must be assured by taking the patient or client to a quiet room or place in the ward where there is no risk of other people over-hearing and minimal chance of being interrupted, and the nurse should convey an impression of being relaxed and unhurried. People will only be able to answer any kind of question fully and openly if they feel secure and think that the listener is genuinely interested in them and what they have to say. A warm, smiling approach and sympathetic, active listening skills are vital in all history-taking, but especially when sexual topics are to be included.

Questions should be framed so as to be meaningful to the patient or client and to encourage a comprehensive answer. Non-directive or open questions such as 'How do you feel about...?' and 'How does that affect you?' will yield more information than closed questions calling only for a 'yes' or 'no' answer, such as 'Are you happy about...?' or 'That makes you feel ill, does it?' Language used in questioning should be appropriate to the listener's level of

1. How has your health/illness affected :–
      your life in general
      your home life
      your work
      how you spend your free time
      how you feel about yourself
      how you get on with other people
      your periods
      your sex life?
2. How has your hospitalisation/treatment/drugs affected:–
      your life in general
      your home life
      your work
      how you spend your free time
      how you feel about yourself
      how you get on with other people
      your periods
      your sex life?
3. Most of us have some religious or other beliefs about relationships, marriage, families, and so on. What beliefs like this are important to you?
4. People often hear stories or half-truths about sexual matters. Have you heard anything like this?
5. Do you have any worries about your health/illness/treatment and its effect on your personal life or your sex life?
6. People often have questions they would like to ask about the sexual side of life. Is there anything you would like to ask?
7. Do you use any kind of contraception? Are you happy with this?
8. Is there anything else at all that you would like to ask or to tell me about? If you think of anything later, do mention it to me or anyone else you feel can help.

Additional questions to be asked for each problem mentioned
Description of problem: Could you tell me a little more about that?
Onset of problem: When did that first happen?
Development or progress: What happened after that?
      How long did it last?
      Did anything make it better?
      Did anything make it worse?
Perception of cause: What do you think was the cause of that?
Expectations for treatment: How do you think people can help you with that?

Figure 10.2 Guidelines for a nursing history about sexuality

understanding, and terminology used in replies should be accepted even when not framed in terms that the nurse would use personally. Therefore, it is important to know colloquialisms, but it is probably better for a nurse not to use them as a matter of course, but only if the interviewee does not appear to understand what is asked (Hogan 1980). Patients will not usually expect nurses to use slang terms and they may lose confidence and regard this as unprofessional. By using neutral terminology nurses teach patients to express themselves, so that they can feel more comfortable in medical encounters through using acceptable language, and emotionally-charged topics are made safer by this means. Euphemisms should be avoided and clarification requested when patients use them, so that answers are correctly interpreted (Lion 1982). Examples of euphemisms which are commonly used but are ambiguous in meaning include 'sleeping' with someone, and 'being careful'. Potentially threatening or embarrassing questions can be 'unloaded' by preceding them with a general statement like 'Many people feel... how about you?' Questioning methods like this avoid the pitfall of conveying assumptions about the interviewee, for not everyone is heterosexual, has genital intercourse, or is sexually active (Woods 1984).

There are many useful books for nurses about communication skills, and further guidance in developing history-taking skills can be learned by reading these. Some examples are included in the list of further reading at the end of this book.

PROBLEMS AND GOALS

A systematic nursing assessment allows patients' problems to be identified, an order of priorities to be decided, and realistic, measurable goals to be established. Most commonly, the problems concerning sexuality which emerge from a nursing history will involve lack of information, belief in incorrect information, or failure of communications between patients or clients and their associates, or between professionals and patients or clients. Only in rare instances will nurses identify actual sexual problems requiring referral to a specialist in sex therapy. As the principal problems are information deficit, misinformation and communications failures, it follows that the goals of nursing care in relation to sexuality will be that patients or clients will receive information and that communications will be improved. Expressing goals in measurable terms and from the patient's or client's point of view requires the use of words and phrases which indicate that information has been received and understood, for example

will repeat information accurately
will explain X in own words
will ask meaningful questions.

Another kind of goal to be achieved by teaching is that a learner is able to use the information gained, and then appropriate and measurable goals could be in the form

makes plans to. . .
chooses to. . .
carries our care
asks nurses/doctors for. . .

If information-giving is designed to reduce anxiety caused by misinformation or lack of information, then possible goals are

says s/he feels happier about X
says s/he is less apprehensive about X
physical signs of anxiety are reduced,
  e.g. pulse rate falls to below 70 per minute
    stops fidgetting with bedclothes
    relaxes facial muscles
    stops biting finger-nails

Goals to be achieved when problems involve communications breakdown involve attempts to start communications flowing freely again by a patient or client initiating a discussion or being receptive to another person's attempt to do so. Once problems are identified, priorities established, and goals set, the appropriate kind of nursing intervention must be chosen and the nursing role which is most likely to lead to goal achievement must be selected.

NURSING INTERVENTIONS

All nurses should be sufficiently knowledgeable about sexuality to take a nursing assessment which includes questions about this area, identify problems, decide what kind of intervention is needed, and evaluate the results of their care. All nurses cannot be sex therapists because this is a highly specialised role, requiring a long period of training and supervised practice (Weinberg 1982, Lion 1982, Woods 1984). A very few patients or clients will be in need of such specialised referral, but many will need information, counselling, or simply an opportunity to talk to a good listener who will not make judgements or criticise while they voice their concerns and work out their own solutions.

Nurses have roles at different levels in relation to sexuality, as Figure 10.3 illustrates, and they may be the most suitable professionals to help the majority of people. Weinberg believes that

> "Nursing is in a unique position to provide for the sexual health care needs of clients. This care is appropriate to the goals of health promotion and primary prevention in nursing. It allows nurses to function as advocates for clients, and enables them to meet the growing demand for informed, responsible client care."
> (Weinberg 1982)

Talking about sexuality is hard for many people because social mores are not conducive to frank discussion of personal, intimate and possibly threatening subjects, even in families or between sexual partners. It can be easier to 'open up' about feelings or reveal a lack of understanding to a sympathetic stranger, and nurses who are skilled communicators and present a warm and non-judgemental manner can act as *facilitators* for patients and clinics needing to talk about their feelings and problems.

Probably everyone has sexual fantasies and dreams, becomes unexpectedly sexually aroused on occasions, or remembers sexual behaviour in childhood. Although all these and many others are 'normal' in the sense that they happen to everyone at some time or another, many people feel guilty about them, wonder if they are 'perverted', and would never dare to mention their thoughts or past to others. Patients or clients may tell nurses about these kinds of fears or may give hints about their insecurities by asking questions like 'How often should a normal person have sex?' or 'Is it true that you can catch diseases if you masturbate?' Nurses who understand the range of sexual expression which exists in our own and other cultures can *validate* the 'normality' and acceptability of any sexual practice which is freely consented to and pleasurable to participants, and help to lift unnecessary burdens of guilt which can interfere with sexual enjoyment.

Teaching about sexuality is probably the most frequent kind of nursing intervention needed. Giving information is one form of teaching, but is not the only way to teach and is often not effective, as the saying 'Teaching isn't telling, listening isn't learning' reminds us. Skilled teaching about sexuality and any

ROLES FOR ALL NURSES	Facilitator
	Validator
	Teacher
	Counsellor
	Advocate
	Referral agent
SPECIALIST ROLE	Sex therapist

Figure 10.3 Nursing roles in relation to sexuality

other subject is based on knowledge about how to structure information in a way most likely to lead to remembering, how to use different teaching methods according to the topic being taught, how visual aids can improve understanding, and a great number of other techniques which can be learned from specialised books. A good example of a book on teaching written especially for nurses is *The Process of Patient Teaching in Nursing Care* by Redman (1980) and full details of this and other books about teaching for nurses are given in the reading list at the end of this book.

Counselling is another special skill which nurses need for all facets of their work, but never more so than in relation to sexuality. Counselling is diametrically opposite to giving people advice about what they should or should not do, and has been defined by the Royal College of Nursing as

"a process through which one person helps another by purposeful conversation in an understanding atmosphere. It seeks to establish a helping relationship in which the one counselled can express his thoughts and feelings in such a way as to clarify his situation, come to terms with some new experiences, see his difficulty more objectively and so face his problem with less anxiety and tension. Its basic purpose is to assist the individual to make his own decision from among the choices available to him."
(Royal College of Nursing 1978)

Counselling about sexuality may be an extension of validating feelings of 'normality'. It may focus, for example, on sexual development at a particular stage in the life cycle, relationships and sexuality, or a whole range of issues including coping with the sexual implications of illness, disability or treatment. Books to help nurses develop skills in counselling are included in the reading list at the end of this book.

The role of *patient advocate* is based on the belief that patients have the right to their own beliefs and convictions, to have their personal dignity and integrity upheld, to be informed about their conditions and different treatment options, and to be involved in decision-making about their own health (Weinberg 1982). In practice, this nursing role includes giving information to patients, ensuring their needs for privacy and confidentiality are met, and involving them in decisions about nursing care. But the advocate role may go beyond these levels to explaining the risks involved in treatments, supporting patients who wish to question other professionals about their treatment, or acting on behalf of patients with their consent to ensure that they receive informed, respectful and humane care (Ashley 1980). Examples of nurses playing an advocate role include informing a women that she is not obliged to agree to a mastectomy if she would rather have a 'lumpectomy', explaining about possible drug side-effects and suggesting that a patient discusses an alternative prescription with the doctor, arranging for a doctor to call back after a round because a patient wishes to have a private talk, or pointing out to a doctor that a patient was embarrassed or distressed by her/his manner or behaviour.

These suggestions may appear to be 'overstepping the mark' in a health care system like ours which has developed on the basis of medical control, and where nurses have usually acted as advocates for doctors rather than patients (Connors 1980), but professionals are above all accountable to their clients. Learning to handle situations where conflict might arise is important for nurses when they are helping to solve patients' problems and also in encounters with colleagues, both in nursing and in other health care professions. Being assertive, and avoiding aggression on the one hand and passivity on the other, is a skill which can be learned, and which can make a valuable contribution towards self-fulfillment in a profession like nursing where social stereotypes and sex-role expectations have been so influential both historically and today. A useful book for both women and men about assertiveness skills is *A Woman in Your Own Right*, by Ann Dickson (1982).

Nurses who detect sexual problems while caring for patients and clients can act as *referral agents* by formally initiating referral to another professional or by giving information about self-help groups, voluntary organisations or educational facilities which may be able to provide the help and support needed. Nurses already refer patients or clients to organisations like the Ileostomy

Association and the Mastectomy Association, which not only deal with practical matters like appliances and diet, but also have experienced counsellors who can offer support over a wide range of areas including sexuality. Family planning clinics are another referral agency recommended by nurses, but there are many lesser-known organisations from SPOD (Sexual and Personal Relationships of the Disabled) to OPUS (Organisations for Parents Under Stress) and Gemma, a support group for lesbians with and without disabilities. A resource list of organisations and groups working in areas related to sexuality is included at the end of this book.

EVALUATION OF CARE

Methods of evaluation of care directed towards sexuality depend on the goals previously established, as with all nursing evaluation. If the goals have been specified clearly and in measurable terms, evaluation follows almost automatically. By comparing patient outcomes with goals, the nurse can decide whether the patient has understood the information given, acted on the knowledge gained, achieved an improvement in symptoms or reached other kinds of specified goals. If the goal has been only partly achieved, not achieved at all, or new problems have arisen since the last assessment, then re-assessment is needed to set revised goals and choose alternative interventions (Kratz 1979). The evaluation stage of the nursing process is thus identical whether the problem being tackled is related to sexuality or any other area of life.

SEXUALITY AND ACTIVITIES OF LIVING

The Activities of Living model of nursing, developed by Roper and her colleagues from Virginia Henderson's work, conceptualises 'Expressing Sexuality' as one of twelve activities of living (Roper, Logan & Tierney 1980). If this model is used as the basis for nursing, the questions relating to sexuality given in Figure 10.2 can be used to collect data when carrying out a nursing assessment. A nursing assessment and care plan based on this model will be described to illustrate how this may be done.

The client whose care will be described is Mrs May Rose, a 73-year-old widow who has lived alone in her ground floor flat since her husband died 4 years ago. Mrs Rose's closest relative is her sister, who lives with her own family in a town 20 miles away, but they are not in close contact because Mrs Rose does not have a telephone. The client has been referred to the district nurse because she was discharged from hospital a week ago, having regained some degree of independence following a right hemisphere cerebrovascular accident. She has been left with mild left-sided hemiplegia, and the district nurse has been asked to check on how she is managing at home.

The Activities of Living model was chosen as the basis for Mrs Rose's assessment (Figure 10.4) and care plan (Figure 10.5) because its underlying philosophy is one of assisting people to regain the maximum independence of which they are capable, and this is precisely what this client has been striving for in hospital and will continue to do at home. The role of the nurse is to assist her in maximising her potential, and the assessment highlights Mrs Rose's outstanding problems in this respect. Independence is an aspect of sexuality, and ability to carry out housekeeping tasks is an important expectation of women in our culture. Personal appearance is another part of sexuality, indicating to others how a person sees herself as a sexual being. Again, our culture has different expectations for women and men, and femininity is defined for many people by an attractive appearance. Post-stroke depression has revived feelings of grief and loss over the death of her husband 4 years ago, and this depression will in turn influence her bowel habits, appetite, dissatisfaction with her physical appearance, and desire to resume her social contacts.

The goals which the district nurse has selected for Mrs Rose involve assisting her return to previous levels of independence by improving her standard of personal hygiene so that she feels more positive about her body image, her depression begins to lift, and she becomes interested in resuming her social activities. In the short term, measures are taken to give her a rapid boost in self-esteem, including helping her to wash her hair. Also in the short term, meals-on-wheels are to be provided on some days to help her to have a nourishing diet while she awaits an occupational therapist's assessment of how she may be aided to cook safely again. This interim measure also aims to give her time to become interested in returning to her lunch club. A possible drug side-effect affecting sexuality is identified, information given to the client about this, and steps taken to deal with the problem. Goal attainment is to be evaluated in two weeks' time, which is intended to be long enough to allow time for some improvements but short enough for any lack of progress not to be damaging.

MAINTAINING A SAFE ENVIRONMENT

Lives alone. Is able to wash at basin but not take a bath for fear of slipping. Cannot cook safely because cooking utensils are too heavy to lift since her stroke has left her with a left-sided weakness. Cooked a hot meal for herself most days before her stroke.

COMMUNICATING

Talks quietly and in short sentences. Appears mildly depressed. Hearing and vision normal.

BREATHING

Respirations: 20 per minute. Blood pressure: 150/85. No problems.

EATING AND DRINKING

Weight 50 kgs on discharge from hospital. Since coming home her usual daily intake is:

> Breakfast – cornflakes, cup of tea
> Mid-morning – cup of tea, 2 biscuits
> Lunch – cheese sandwich, jam tart, cup of tea
> Mid-afternoon – cup of tea
> Tea – meat-paste sandwich, cake, cup of tea
> Night drink – tea

Has one pint of milk every other day. See MAINTAINING A SAFE ENVIRONMENT

ELIMINATING

No urinary problems. Constipated: used to have a daily bowel action but now this only occurs every 2–3 days and with difficulty. See EATING AND DRINKING.

PERSONAL CLEANSING AND DRESSING

See MAINTAINING A SAFE ENVIRONMENT. Can dress herself slowly, uses garters to hold up stockings. Cannot reach up with left arm so is unable to wash her hair. Is distressed about this and feels she looks unattractive and dirty. Would like to go to a hairdresser but cannot afford it.

Figure 10.4 Nursing assessment of Mrs Rose, based on the Roper Activities of Living Model

The definition which forms the basis for this book conceptualises sexuality as an integral part of total personhood and life-style. The fact that sexuality touches so many areas of life made it difficult to decide where data should be placed on the Activities of Living assessment form. For example, Mrs Rose's distress about her *continued*

CONTROLLING BODY TEMPERATURE

No problems. Flat has a gas fire in living room and she has an electric fire and electric blanket in bedroom.

MOBILISING

Is moving slowly but efficiently despite left hemiplegia. Is right-handed. Goes to local shops and can carry small amounts of shopping.

WORKING AND PLAYING

Feels lonely since coming out of hospital. Sister lives too far to visit, and neighbours are out at work all day. Used to go to Lunch Club at Neighbourhood Centre three times a week, and enjoyed talking to one particular man there. Does not want to go now because of her unwashed hair. Can dust and tidy flat, and make bed (has a duvet). Can put small items in washing machine, but cannot hang things on the line to dry, and cannot iron.

EXPRESSING SEXUALITY

Feels her stroke has changed her life a great deal and is worried about her future independence. Stroke has stopped her cooking, going out to her club, bathing and keeping up her appearance as she would like. Misses the company of people at the Lunch Club. Has had several tearful spells in the evenings because she feels lonely and unwanted, and is thinking a lot about her husband who died 4 years ago. *NB* Is taking anti-hypertensive drugs.

SLEEPING

Has difficulty getting off to sleep, and wakes at about 5 a.m. and cannot go back to sleep. Averages 5–6 hours of sleep per night but does not feel tired because she is not being very active. Used to sleep 7 hours per night, but is not worried about sleeping.

DYING

Feels she has been lucky to have such a mild stroke and still be able to stay in her own flat. Knows she could have another stroke and must take her 'blood pressure tablets'. Says she would rather die if she had another stroke, and not have to 'go into a home'.

deteriorating appearance is an aspect of Expressing Sexuality, but also of Personal Cleansing and Hygiene, and Working and Playing. This meant that a certain amount of repetition was unavoidable if the assessment form was to be comprehensively completed. The same problem arose when writing the care plan, but unneces-

Figure 10.5 Nursing care plan for Mrs Rose, based on the Roper Activities of Living Model

PROBLEMS Actual & Potential	GOALS	INTERVENTIONS	DATE FOR EVALUATION
MAINTAINING A SAFE ENVIRONMENT			
P Accident with saucepans if she tries to cook	Will be able to cook safely	Discuss risks with patient. Request assessment by occupational therapist regarding aids and modifications to kitchen and bathroom	2 weeks
P Accident if she tries to get into bath	Will be able to bath safely		
EATING AND DRINKING			
A Unable to cook and therefore is not having a balanced diet	*Short term* Improve nutrition by having meals on wheels 3 times weekly *Long term* Will return to Lunch Club and to cooking for herself	Suggest meals on wheels as a purely temporary solution. Order meals for Mondays, Wednesdays and Fridays	2 weeks
P Loss of weight (is already 3 kgs underweight for height)	Will maintain present weight or gain weight	Advise on diet for days when she does not have meals on wheels. Recommend suitable protein and fibre-rich foods which are cheap and easy to prepare, e.g. cheese, fresh fruit. See ELIMINATING	2 weeks

ELIMINATING

A Constipation due to lack of fibre in diet	Will return to having a daily bowel action	Give leaflet on high fibre foods, go through it with her and suggest suitable daily intake	2 weeks

PERSONAL CLEANSING AND DRESSING

A Cannot get into bath	Will be able to have a bath	See MAINTAINING A SAFE ENVIRONMENT. Advise to have an all-over wash at the basin while awaiting assessment for aids	2 weeks
A Cannot wash her hair	Hair will be washed weekly. Will say she feels happy with her hair	Help her to wash her hair today. Investigate facilities at Neighbourhood Centre for hair-washing, and concessions for pensioners at local hairdressers	

WORKING AND PLAYING

A Feels lonely and isolated since she has stopped going to club	Will start going to club again	See PERSONAL CLEANSING AND HYGIENE	2 weeks
A Unable to do heavier housework since stroke	*Short term* Will have assistance with housework *Long term* Will regain independence with housework	Arrange home help one morning per week to do heavier jobs and shopping while awaiting occupational therapy assessment	2 weeks

Continued overleaf

PROBLEMS	GOALS	INTERVENTIONS	DATE FOR EVALUATION
EXPRESSING SEXUALITY			
A Feels unattractive and thinks other people will not want to be close to her	Will say she feels happy with her appearance and hygiene. Will return to club	See PERSONAL CLEANSING AND HYGIENE Investigate possibility of some of friends from club calling round to see her when she is ready for this	2 weeks
A Mildly depressed due to stroke and loss of independence, possibly made worse by anti-hypertensive drugs	Will say her tearful spells are less and will express interest in going to club	Encourage her to express her feelings by active listening, non-verbal communication, and open-ended questions. Explain that depression often occurs after a stroke, that she will feel better as she regains her independence, and that her blood pressure tablets may be making things worse. Tell her you will ask her GP to review the position but that she should continue to take the tablets in the meantime. Inform GP that patient is de-pressed and ask her to reassess patient	

DYING

A Pessimistic view of Will say she feels more See PERSONAL CLEANSING 2 weeks
  her future due to loss independent again   AND DRESSING and EXPRESS-
  of independence and Will return to club   ING SEXUALITY
  self-esteem following
  stroke

P Stopping   anti- Will continue to take See EXPRESSING SEXUALITY 2 weeks
  hypertensive drugs drugs or an alternative
  due to side-effects prescribed by GP
  and lack of interest in
  prolonging her life

sary repetition was avoided by referring back to previous sections rather than rewriting items. Time is an important consideration when writing care plans, and a method is required which allows the maximum time to be devoted to patient care rather than excessive documentation. Therefore, it seems justified to use ways of saving time by not repeating items when this does not sacrifice clarity and completeness.

An approach which is adopted by some who use this model, is to reserve the 'Expressing Sexuality' section of the assessment form for information directly or indirectly concerning reproduction, such as menstruation, engorged breasts and maternal bonding. Others make very little use of this section, whether from lack of understanding of the complexities of sexuality or because of difficulty in deciding how to record information. These strategies either reduce the concept of sexuality to a more or less biological one, or ignore it altogether. Roper *et al.* (1983) are aware of these difficulties but see no way to modify the model to take account of them. Although repetition is time-consuming, it is surely preferable to omission of important information and neglect of problems, and the solutions adopted in Mrs Reid's care plan therefore seem justifiable.

SEXUALITY AND ADAPTATION

In Roy's Adaptation Model, a human being is defined as a biopsychosocial system which is in constant interaction with the external environment, and whose internal subsystems are also in constant change (Riehl & Roy 1980). People use both innate and acquired mechanisms to adapt to the stimuli or stressors encountered in these changing environments. Nursing is concerned with manipulating these stimuli to assist people to make adaptations and thereby to move towards the peak wellness extreme of a continuum which stretches from peak wellness through poor health to death at the other extreme.

People have four modes or subsystems which can adapt, according to Roy's model. The *physiological* subsystem includes exercise and rest, nutrition, elimination, fluid and electrolytes, oxygen, circulation and regulation. The *self-concept* subsystem is the self which responds to environmental changes, the *role function* subsystem regulates the performance of duties in various social roles, and the *interdependence* subsystem involves interaction between individuals and others. All four modes or subsystems interact with and influence each other, making up the totality of a person.

Three kinds of stimuli or stressors affecting people's levels of adaptation are envisaged by the model. A *focal* stimulus is the immediate cause of a problem or stress, *contextual* stimuli are other stressors present in the environment, while *residual* stimuli are beliefs, attitudes, characteristics and experiences which arise from past experience.

A nursing assessment carried out using the Roy model has two levels. Firstly, behaviours in the four modes of adaptation are assessed to identify deviations from normality. Then, a second level assessment concentrates on identifying the focal, contextual and residual stimuli causing the health-deviation or stress, so that nursing interventions can be directed towards manipulating these stimuli and helping the individual to adapt or make a positive response (Rambo 1984).

The patient whose care has been planned using the Roy Adaptation Model is John House, a 53-year-old married man who is a self-employed taxi driver. He lives with his wife, Betty, who is a full-time housewife, and their son (aged 20) and daughter (18 years old) who are both students. John had a myocardial infarction a week ago and his obesity, sedentary life-style and financial strains doubtless played a causal role in this (Macleod 1981).

His nursing assessment (Figure 10.6) and teaching plan (Figure 10.7) are based on the Roy model, which was chosen because John needs to make some fundamental changes or adaptations in his life-style if he is to regain his health and avoid another heart attack. John has a low degree of understanding about the influence of his life-style in leading to his heart attack, and sees his masculinity as closely tied in with his role as family breadwinner and decision-taker. He is unaccustomed to being other than independent and in control of his life, and finds it hard to see that he needs to share responsibilities and allow others to help him. Therefore a teaching plan has been drawn up to give John the information he needs and to encourage him to use this information to adapt to his new situation and involve his family in supporting him.

Sexuality is not specifically mentioned in the Roy assessment scheme, but a knowledge of the subject allows the nurse to be alert

Figure 10.6 Nursing assessment of John House, based on the Roy Adaptation Model

FIRST LEVEL ASSESSMENT	SECOND LEVEL ASSESSMENT		
	FOCAL STIMULI	CONTEXTUAL STIMULI	RESIDUAL STIMULI
BASIC PHYSIOLOGICAL NEEDS			
Exercise and rest	Sleeps from 1 a.m. to 6.30 a.m., dozes in taxi for an hour in the afternoon if not busy	Working hours long, starts early and ends late	Pressures of self-employment and supporting family	Cultural values associated with masculinity and being head of family
Nutrition	10kgs overweight for height. Eats a fried breakfast, take-away lunch eaten in taxi, goes home for evening meal	Overweight	Stress and working hours make it hard to have a balanced diet	Men do not usually learn much about food and cooking
Elimination	Bowels opened regularly. No problems with micturition	No problems		
Fluid and electrolytes	Drinks canned soft drinks while working, and a 'large Scotch' at night to help him sleep	Overweight	Job makes it hard to take breaks for drinks	

Oxygen	Gets breathless if he runs, carries heavy objects, etc. 'I'm not as young as I used to be'. Used to smoke 30 cigarettes daily but gave up 3 years ago	Breathless on ex-ertion	Overweight and used to smoke heavily	Used to smoke heavily. Cultural values of ambition and financial success for men
Circulation	No apparent problems prior to heart attack	Has had a myocardial infarction	Stressful life-style, excess and unbalanced diet, lack of exercise	
Regulation a. Temperature b. Senses c. Endocrine system	37.2°C Normal Normal	No problems No problems No problems		

SELF-CONCEPT

1. Physical self	Says he's 'always been a big man'	Overweight	Associates masculinity with being physically big	Cultural definitions of masculinity and strength
2. Personal self a. moral-eth-ical-guilt	Feels guilty that he has had to take time off work. Family will suffer financially as he is the only wage-earner	Has had a myocardial infarction	Hospitalisation and need to rest Financial worries	As above

Continued overleaf

FIRST LEVEL ASSESSMENT	FOCAL STIMULI	CONTEXTUAL STIMULI	RESIDUAL STIMULI
b. self-consistency-anxiety	Is worried that his heart attack may stop him working. Has heard that men have to stop having sex after a heart attack because it can cause another attack. Says his sex life 'isn't what it used to be' anyway because he is always tired and gets breathless	As above	Threat of not being able to work as before. Fear that sex life is at an end	Cultural stereotypes of sexuality and gender roles
c. self-ideal and expectancy – powerlessness	Feels depressed that his whole life may have to change and he will be an invalid	As above	Feels responsible for his family. Wife does not work and children are at college. Feels he should earn enough to support them.	As above
3. Interpersonal self				
a. social disengagement	Does not want to talk to his wife about his condition and its implications	As above	Not used to talking about problems and resents the need to do so now	As above

b. aggression	Has had an argument with his wife because she made suggestions about how they could manage financially and how he could adapt his work routine	As above	Reluctant to appear weak and to listen to advice	As above
ROLE FUNCTION				
a. role failure	Feels he will no longer be a 'real man' if he cannot support his family and help his children through college	As above	Feelings of potential failure as a male, husband and father	As above
b. role conflict	Thinks he will have to change his work routine but needs to earn as much as he can	As above	As above	
INTERDEPENDENCE	Has always been the breadwinner and decision-maker. 'They look up to me', 'I'm a very independent man', 'I've never asked anyone for anything'	As above	Not used to asking for help or not being able to manage alone. Does not share his feelings with others	As above

Figure 10.7 Teaching plan for John House, based on the Roy Adaptation Model

PROBLEM	GOAL	INTERVENTION	EVALUATION CRITERIA
Need for adaptations in life-style after heart attack	Will understand the role of life-style in causing heart attacks	Sit down with John and his wife and to go through booklet 'After Your Heart Attack'. Give John his own copy to read and take home for reference.	John and his wife discuss information in booklet and ask relevant questions. *John* reads through booklet alone later
	Will begin to discuss with wife and family adaptations in life-style	Focus on one topic in the booklet each day, relate it specifically to John and explain that:– – he will be given an Out Patient appointment for 6 weeks' time. Until then he should not work, but gently increase his activities according to how he feels and tiredness levels, avoiding activities which cause pain or breathlessness – GTN tablets should be	*John, his wife and children:–* – discuss his convalescence together and with nurse, and ask questions to help in making plans – tell nurses about plans to help John during his recovery *John:–* – takes GTN tablets when required – asks if he may go for a walk outside the ward – talks optimistically

placed under the tongue before taking exercise which may cause anginal pain
- doctor will advise at OP appointment about return to work. When he is ready to work, shorter hours would be advisable
- walking on fairly level ground is a good form of exercise to build up strength. Regular exercise within comfort limits is part of prevention of further problems
- sex is not an especially hazardous activity. When he is able to walk up 2 flights of stairs comfortably, he is ready for sexual activity if he wishes. Sex and all strenuous activity should be avoided after a heavy meal, after drinking alcohol, when tired or under stress

about his convalescence and future lifestyle
- says he feels ready to manage at home

Continued overleaf

PROBLEM	GOAL	INTERVENTION	EVALUATION CRITERIA
Obesity	Will eat a balanced, nutritious diet appropriate to his activity levels	Explain the role of diet in health and its link with heart disease	Repeats explanation accurately and ask further questions
	Short-term Accepts a dietary assessment	Ask John to see a dietician for assessment and counselling	John says he would like to see the dietician
		Arrange dietician's visit for one afternoon when Mrs House will be visiting	
	Choose suitable foods from hospital menu	After dietician's visit, help John to choose his meals from the menu, using the diet sheet given to him by dietician for guidance	Consults leaflet and orders appropriate meals

Does not cheat on his diet	Suggest John asks his wife to take the Lucozade and biscuits home and bring him some low calorie fruit juice and fruit	Has no biscuits or high calorie drinks on his locker, but has fruit and low calorie drinks instead
	Suggest he keeps a diary of what he eats, and discusses this with dietician or nurses	Discusses intake with dietician or nurse, points out where he has 'cheated' and where diary shows progress towards better diet
Begins to lose weight	Give John a weight chart and show him how to record his weight weekly	Records weight accurately and achieves a drop in weight
Long-term Aim for a weight loss of 10kgs in 3 months	Show John weight and height tables and agree a target weight	Weight loss of 10kgs in 3 months (to be evaluated on Out Patient visits after discharge)

to points which link with sexuality. These points occur mainly in the self-concept subsystem, where sexuality both contributes to and results from the way individuals see themselves, in the role function subsystem because social roles build identity and self-esteem, and in the interdependence subsystem where relationships with others help people to define and value themselves. Roy's model is not clear about which items of information should be placed in which subsystem and, as we have seen throughout this book, it would probably be impossible to make such a neat separation because self-concept, roles and relationships are part of the totality of a person, each influencing the other. This failure to be clear about definitions of the subsystems is an inadequacy of the Roy model. Nevertheless, using the model to plan John's care provided a systematic framework for identifying problems and indicating where interventions should be focussed.

CONCLUSION

In this chapter we have seen how nurses can use knowledge and understanding of sexuality throughout the nursing process to achieve a holistic approach to care. Two examples have illustrated how sexuality is incorporated into two different nursing models, with benefits and disadvantages in each case. The models provide a framework for thinking about care, an assessment tool, and a general approach to intervention. But they are based on 'high level' theories and a great deal of 'middle level' knowledge is needed to add flesh to their skeletons so that care is comprehensively planned, given and evaluated. The 'middle level' knowledge used to compile the two care plans concerned sexuality itself, information about causes of illness, social services available in the community, and theories of teaching and counselling.

In this book, sexuality has been discussed from the perspective of patients and clients, nurses and informal carers. The aim has been to show that sexuality should be a fundamental focus of nursing care in all specialities, and in institutional as well as community care. Sexuality is at the centre of social development at this moment in our culture, as gender stereotypes are increasingly challenged and equal opportunities legislation is beginning to have some effects. In the concluding chapter, links between nursing and social changes today and in the future will be explored in the same way as they were in relation to developments in the past, and once again sexuality will emerge as a key issue for nurses.

CHAPTER 11

Sexuality and Nursing: The Future

Nursing and sexuality have been closely intertwined throughout history, even before Florence Nightingale established nursing as a profession specifically for women in the 19th century. In the early 20th century some nurses played a leading role in the women's suffrage struggle. But the sexuality-nursing link took on a different form when, after the insistence of a separate register for men, and their exclusion from the Royal College of Nursing until 1960, 'masculine' values began to encroach upon nursing management. Following the Salmon Report (HMSO 1966), men became the majority in positions of power in nursing while remaining the minority among nurses as a whole.

Outside nursing, social attitudes and behaviour in the realms of sexuality have been in a state of radical change for the past 25 years. Stereotypes of femininity and masculinity are being broken down in some respects, as make-up, jewellery, shoulder bags and 'unisex' clothes become acceptable for women and men alike. The new model of sexuality is more androgynous, combining variable mixes of what were previously seen as feminine or masculine behavioural styles (Bem 1974), and is represented by such unlikely companions as Boy George, with his long hair and make-up, and women astronauts and prime ministers who do jobs and take decisions reserved for men until very recently. In other ways, social change is paradoxically moving in the opposite direction, with women being encouraged to return to the home and devote themselves exclusively to motherhood and housewifery at a time of economic decline and unemployment.

177

The 'consumer' movement in health is gaining ground as people become more and more dissatisfied with high-tech/low-touch treatment and seek the more humanistic forms of care offered by acupuncture, meditation, herbal remedies and self-help groups. A television in almost every home, as well as longer years of schooling, has raised knowledge and awareness levels about health and health care, with the result that patients and clients want to understand how their bodies work and to participate in decisions about their own treatment. Rising expectations about the quality of care and consumers' rights are therefore confronting health professionals (Haug & Lavin 1981), and patients and clients increasingly want the kind of health care that responds to all their needs. They want to be seen not just as broken-down bodies to be repaired like cars, but as unique individuals with a wide range of needs of which sexuality is one (Holderby & McNulty 1982).

Earlier nurses were influenced by feminist ideas, but today there is a wide gulf separating most nurses from the women's movement (Glass & Brand 1979). The majority of nurses see no connection between their profession and feminist ideas, but feminist nurses argue that there is a very close link between the two. Feminists think that standards of behaviour and opportunities to study and work in demanding and satisfying jobs should not be allocated according to sex, but that both women and men should be free to live and organise their lives as they wish. Women have traditionally been prevented from doing this because society is dominated by men, and many interesting and rewarding opportunities, both emotionally and materially, have been reserved for them. The qualities regarded as 'female', which have defined the caring role of women as wives, mothers and housewives, are more truly 'human' qualities than the hard, rational and emotionally distant model learned by men. Feminists would like to see these 'female' values becoming the dominant ones, and they believe that people would be happier, and women and men would gain more personal fulfillment, if they shared in childcare and were able to choose without restrictions any kind of job they were capable of doing. Ascendance of these 'feminine' values would lead to less aggression and conflict, and therefore war would be much less likely than it is in a society where boys learn to fight at a very young age and to disdain showing and talking about their feelings. Over a long period of time, gender stereotypes would be eroded because children would see their mothers and fathers acting in different ways and they would have alternative role models to imitate. It would be impossible to predict in any detail what this future society would be like, because different ways of socialisation could allow people to develop in ways we have no means of anticipating, and simply to imagine 'masculine' women and 'feminine' men is unduly restricting. Totally new ways of being could unfold for women and men if they were liberated from the restrictions and unfairness of traditional stereotypes (Chodorow 1978).

It is likely that sexuality and nursing will continue to be closely interlinked in the future as they have been in the past, but the nature of the link depends greatly on nurses themselves. Nurses can either remain on a divergent path from wider society, ignoring sexuality in nursing and following stereotyped patterns of behaviour (Glass & Brand 1979). Or they can critically examine evidence, as we have done in this book, decide that personal and professional self-esteem and gratification depend on no longer being bound by crushing stereotypes, and be assertive in securing high quality nursing care through a truly holistic approach which respects the sexuality of all who are involved in the health care system. They can decide that our anatomy should no longer control our destiny as nurses, clients or informal carers, and work to stamp out the infection of inequality in the health care system. If nurses ignore the challenges of social change they are, in doing so, condoning present standards of care and professionalism. As an American nurse has pointed out, this amounts of saying to others, 'Go ahead, I'm behind you... way behind you' (Dean 1982). Is this an acceptable stance for a caring profession?

Useful Addresses

You can often be put in touch with your nearest local contact via these addresses. As these are non-profitmaking organisations, please enclose a stamped and addressed envelope for your reply if you write to them. Telephone numbers are given where there is an emergency line, but not all of these operate a 24-hour service so you may need to try at different times of the day.

BOOKSHOPS

Gay's the Word, 66 Marchmont Street, London WC1
Grassroots Books, 1 Newton Street, Manchester 1
Lavender Menace Bookshop, 11a Forth Street, Edinburgh
Sisterwrite Bookshop, 190 Upper Street, London N1

CONTRACEPTION AND ABORTION

British Pregnancy Advisory Service (BPAS), Airsty Manor, Wootton Warren, Solihull, West Midlands
Brook Advisory Centre, 233 Tottenham Court Road, London W1
Family Planning Information Service, 27–35 Mortimer Street, London W1N 7RJ
Marie Stopes Clinic, 108 Whitfield Street, London W1
Pregnancy Advisory Service (PAS), 40 Margaret Street, London W1
Ulster Pregnancy Advisory Service, 338a Lisburn Road, Belfast.

COUNSELLING

Association of Sexual and Marital Therapists, PO Box 62, Sheffield S10 3TS

British Association for Counselling, 37a Sheep Street, Coventry, Warwickshire CV21 3BX

Catholic Marriage Advisory Council, 15 Lansdown Road, London W11 3AJ

Family Planning Association (for information on sexual counselling services), 27 Mortimer Street, London W1N 7RJ

Identity Counselling Service (for sexual, personal or relationships problems) Beauchamp Lodge, 2 Warwick Close, London W2 6NE

Jewish Marriage Guidance Council, 529b Finchley Road, London NW3 7BG

National Marriage Guidance Council, Herbert Gray College, Little Church Street, Rugby, Warwickshire CV21 3AP

National Association of Young People's Counselling and Advisory Services, 17–23 Albion Street, Leicester LE1 6GD

Northern Ireland Marriage Guidance Council, 76 Dublin Road, Belfast BT2 7HP

Organisation for Parents Under Stress (OPUS), 26 Manor Drive, Pickering, Yorkshire

Samaritans, 01–283–3400 (24-hour service)

Scottish Marriage Guidance Council, 26 Frederick Street, Edinburgh EH2 2JR

Westminster Pastoral Foundation (counselling on relationships and sexuality, 23 Kensington Square, London W8 5HN

GAY AND LESBIAN CENTRES

Birmingham Lesbian and Gay Centre Committee, c/o 40 Thorpe Street, Birmingham 4

Edinburgh Gay Centre, 58a Broughton Street, Edinburgh

Liverpool Gay Centre, 14 Colquitt Street, Liverpool

London Lesbian and Gay Centre, 67–69 Cowcross Street, London EC1

Manchester Gay Centre, 61a Bloom Street, Manchester

GAY RIGHTS AND INFORMATION ORGANISATIONS

Campaign for Homosexual Equality, 24 Upper Street, London N1 2UA

Gay Bereavement Project, Unitarian Rooms, Hoop Lane, London NW11 8BS

Gay Rights Office, National Council for Civil Liberties, 21 Tabard Street, London SE1

GEMMA (for lesbians with/out disabilities), BM Box 5700, London WC1N 3XX

Lesbian Custody Network, Rights of Women, c/o 152 Camden High
   Street, London NW1
Northern Ireland Gay Rights Association, PO Box 44, Belfast BT1 1SH
Parents' Enquiry (for parents with gay daughters or sons) c/o Rose
   Robertson, 16 Honley Road, London SE6 2HZ
Scottish Homosexual Rights Group, 60 Broughton Street, Edinburgh
   EH1 3SA
Terence Higgins Trust (AIDS information service), 38 Mount
   Pleasant Road WC1

MEN'S GROUPS AND SERVICES FOR MEN

Achilles Heel (Men's magazine), 7 St Mark's Rise, London E8
Anti-sexist Men's Newsletter, c/o Misha, 12 Terrapin Road, London
   SW17
London Men's Centre, c/o Bread and Roses, 316 Upper Street,
   London N1

NURSES' ORGANISATIONS

Association of Radical Midwives, 8a The Drive, Wimbledon, London
   SW20
Radical Health Visitors, c/o British Society for Social Responsibility
   in Science, 9 Poland Street, London W1
Radical Nurses' Groups, 20 Melrose Road, Sheffield 3

RAPE CRISIS CENTRES

Aberdeen, PO Box 123. 0224–575560
Belfast, PO Box 46. 0232–249696
Bradford, PO Box 155. 0274–308270
Brighton 0273–699756
Cambridge 0223–358314
Canterbury 0227–50400
Cardiff 022–373181
Cleveland 0642–813397
Coventry 0203–77229
Dublin 0001–601–470
Edinburgh, PO Box 120.
Glasgow, PO Box 53. 041–221–8448
Leeds 0532–44058
Leicester 0536–666666
Liverpool 051–734–4369

London, PO Box 69, London WC1. 01–278–3956
Manchester 061–228–3602
Norwich 0603–667687
Nottingham 0602–410440
Oxford 0865–72695
Portsmouth 0705–669511
Reading 0734–55577
Sheffield, PO Box 34. 0742–755255
Tyneside 0632–329858

SPECIALIST HEALTH, ILLNESS AND DISABLEMENT GROUPS AND ORGA-
NISATIONS

Age Concern, Bernard Sunley House, 60 Pitcairn Road, Mitcham,
  Surrey
Alcoholics Anonymous, 7 Moreton Street, London SW1
*Alcohol Community Centre for Education, Prevention and Treatment
  (ACCEPT),* Western Hospital, Seagrave Road, London SW6
Alcoholism, London Council on, 146 Queen Victoria Street, London
  EC4
Anorexic Aid, c/o Alison Cork, The Priory Centre, 11 Priory Road,
  High Wycombe, Bucks.
Arthritis Care, 6 Grosvenor Crescent, London SW1X 7ER
Cancer Foundation, Ulster (runs a mastectomy advisory service),
  40–42 Eglantine Avenue, Belfast BT9 6DX
Carers, Association of, 58 New Road, Chatham, Kent
Carers and their Dependents, National Council for, 29 Chilworth
  Mews, London W2 3RG
Chest, Heart and Stroke Association, Tavistock House North, Tavis-
  tock Square, London WC1H 9JE
Childless, National Assocation for the, Birmingham Settlement, 318
  Summer Lane, Birmingham B19 3RL
Colostomy Welfare Group, 38–39 Eccleston Square, London SW1V
  1PB
Compulsive Eating Group, c/o Spare Tyre, 86–88 Holmleigh Road,
  London N16
Coronary Prevention Group, Central Middlesex Hospital, Acton
  Lane, London NW10 7NF
Diabetic Association, British, 10 Queen Anne Street, London W1M
  0BD
Disabled Living Foundation, 346 Kensington High Street, London
  W14 8NS
Disabled, Sexual and Personal Relations of the (SPOD), 286 Camden
  Road, London N7 0BJ

Disability Alliance, 1 Cambridge Terrace, London NW1
Disability Income Group, 28 Commercial Street, London W1
Disability and Rehabilitation, Royal Association for (RADAR), 25
  Mortimer Street, London W1N 8AB
Drugs: Release, 1 Elgin Avenue, London W9 3PR. 01–603–8654 (24
  hour service)
Drugs: Tranx, c/o 2 St John's Road, Harrow, Middlesex
Equal Opportunities Commission, Overseas House, Quay Street,
  Manchester 3
Ileostomy Association, Central Office, Amblehurst House,
  Chobham, Woking, Surrey
Incontinence Advisors, Association of, c/o Disabled Living Founda-
  tion, 346 Kensington High Street, London W14 8NS
Mental Health, National Assocation for (MIND), 22 Harley Street,
  London W1N 2ED
Pre-retirement Association, 19 Undine Street, London SW17 8PP
Single parents: Gingerbread, 35 Wellington Street, London WC2
Single parents: National Council for One-Parent Families, 255
  Kentish Town Road, London NW5 2LX
Smoking and Health, Action on (ASH), 5–11 Mortimer Street, Lon-
  don W1
Spina Bifida and Hydrocephalus, Association for, Tavistock House
  North, Tavistock Square, London WC1 9JH
Spinal Injuries Association, 5 Crowndale Road, London NW1
Urinary Conduit Association, 8 Coniston Close, Dane Bank, Denton,
  Manchester M34 2EW

WOMEN'S HEALTH AND SELF-HELP GROUPS

Alcohol Centre, Women's, 254 St Paul's Road, London N1
Alcohol: Drugs, Alcohol Women Nationally (DAWN), c/o London
  Council on Alcoholism, 146 Queen Victoria Street, London EC4
Assertiveness training: Redwood Women's Association, 83 Ford-
  wych Road, London NW2
Cancer Control Campaign, Women's National, 1 South Audley Street,
  London W1Y 5DQ
Counselling Centre, Oxford Women's, Highcroft House, Tanners
  Lane, Off Queen Street, Eynsham, Oxon
Cystitis: U & I Club, 18 Southcote Way, Tylers Green, Bucks
Disablement, Sisters Against (SAD), 54 Whitby Court, Parkhurst
  Road, London N7 0SU
Drugs, Alcohol Women Nationally (DAWN), c/o London Council on
  Alcoholism, 146 Queen Victoria Street, London EC4

Endometriosis Self-help Group, c/o Ailsa Irving, 65 Holmdene Avenue, London SE24 9LD

Health Concern, Women's (For advice on where to seek help), 16 Seymour Street, London W1H 5WB

Health Information Centre, Women's (WHIC), 53 Featherstone Street, London EC1

Health Shop, Women's, 32 High Street, Edinburgh EH1 1TB

Hysterectomy Support Group, c/o Judy Vaughan, Rivendell, Warren Way, Lower Heswall, Wirral, Merseyside

Information, Referral and Enquiries Service, Women's (WIRES), 32a Shakespeare Street, Nottingham. Phone-in information service 0602–411476

Mastectomy Association of Great Britain, 25 Brighton Road, Croydon, Surrey

Miscarriage Association, 2 West Vale, Thornhill Road, Dewsbury, West Yorks WF12 9QH

Pelvic Inflammatory Disease Self-help Group, c/o Jessica Pickard, 32 Parkholme Road, London E8

Therapy Centre, Women's, 6 Manor Gardens, London N7

Therapy Centre, Pellin South London Feminist, 43 Killyon Road, London SW8

Work Hazards Group, Women and, c/o British Society for Social Responsibility in Science, 9 Poland Street, London W1

WOMEN'S AID (REFUGES FOR BATTERED WOMEN)

English National Office, 374 Gray's Inn Road, London WC1 (01–837–9316 (24-hour service)

Northern Ireland National Office, 134 University Street, Belfast 7. 02327–249378

Scottish National Office, 11 St Colme Street, Edinburgh. 031–225–8011

Welsh National Office, Incentive House, Adams Street, Cardiff. 0222–388291

References and Further Reading

Altman D (1973) *Homosexual*. London: Penguin

Archer J & Lloyd B (1982) *Sex and Gender*. Harmondsworth: Penguin

Ashley J A (1980) Power in structured misogyny: implications for the politics of care. *Advances in Nursing Science*, **2**(3), 3–22

Austin R (1977) Sex and Gender in the future of nursing 1. *Nursing Times*, Occasional Papers, **73**(34), 113–116

Austin R (1977) Sex and gender in the future of nursing 2. *Nursing Times*, Occasional Papers **73**(35), 117–119

Barrett M & McIntosh M (1982) *The Anti-social Family*. London: Verso

Bart P (1971) Depression in middle-aged women. *Women in Sexist Society*, ed V Gornick & B Moran. New York: Basic Books

Bartels E (1982) Biological sex differences and sex stereotyping. *The Changing Experience of Women*, ed E Whitelegg *et al.* Oxford: Martin Robertson/Open University

Beck A (1968) *Depression*. New York: Harper & Row

Beechey V (1983) *The Changing Experience of Women. Units 10 & 11. Women and Employment*. Milton Keynes: Open University

Beechey V & Allen R (1982) *The Changing Experience of Women. Unit 1. The Woman Question*. Milton Keynes: Open University

Bem S (1974) The measurement of psychological androgyny. *Journal of Consulting & Clinical Psychology*, **42**, 155–162

Biller H B (1976) Paternal deprivation and sex-role development. *The Role of the Father in Child Development*, ed M E Lamb. New York: J Wiley

Bingham S (1979) *Ministering Angels*. London: Osprey

Birke L & Gardner K (1979) *Why Suffer? Periods and their Problems*. London: Virago

Birke L *et al* eds (1980) *Alice through the Looking Glass*. London: Virago

Bridge W & MacLeod Clark J (1981) *Communication in Nursing Care*. Chichester: HM&M Publishers/Wiley

Brookfield G, Douglas A, Shapiro R S & Cias S J (1982) Some thoughts on being a male in nursing. *Socialisation, Sexism and Stereotyping. Women's Issues in Nursing,* ed J Muff. St Louis: C V Mosby

Brown G W & Harris T (1978) *The Social Origins of Depression.* London: Tavistock Publications

Brown P ed (1973) *Radical Psychology.* New York: Harper & Row

Brownmiller S (1975) *Against Our Will. Men, Women and Rape.* Harmondsworth: Penguin

Bush M A & Kjervik D K (1979) The nurse's self-image. *Women in Stress: A Nursing Perspective,* ed D K Kjervik & I M Martinson. New York: Appleton-Century-Crofts

Byrne E M (1978) *Women and Education.* London: Tavistock Publications

Cannedy N N (1979) Florence Nightingale: woman with a vision. *Women in Stress: A Nursing Perspective,* ed D K Kjervik & I M Martinson. New York: Appleton-Century-Crofts

Carpenter M (1977) The new managerialism and professionalism in nursing. *Health and the Division of Labour,* ed M Stacey, M Reid, C Heath & R Dingwall. London: Croom Helm

Carver V & Liddiard P eds (1978) *An Ageing Population.* Sevenoaks: Hodder & Stoughton/Open University

Charlesworth A, Wilkin D & Durie A (1984) *Carers and Services: A Comparison of Men and Women Caring for Dependent and Elderly People.* Manchester: Equal Opportunities Commission

Chesler P (1972) *Women and Madness.* London: Allen Lane

Chodorow N (1978) *The Reproduction of Mothering. Psychoanalysis and the Sociology of Gender.* Berkeley: University of California Press

Cockburn C (1977) *The Local State.* London: Pluto Press

Cohen F & Lazarus R (1973) Active coping processes, coping dispositions, and recovery from surgery. *Psychosomatic Medicine,* **35,** 375–389

Comfort A (1977) *A Good Age.* London: Beasley

Comfort A (1975) *The Joy of Sex.* London: Penguin

Connors D D (1980) Sickness unto death: medicine as mythic, necrophilic and iatrogenic. *Advances in Nursing Science,* **2**(3), 39–51

Counter Information Services (1981) *Women in the 80s.* London: Counter Information Services

Curran L (1980) Science education: did she drop out or was she pushed? *Alice Through the Looking Glass,* ed L Birke et al. London: Virago

Danziger K ed (1970) *Readings in Child Socialisation.* New York: Pergamon

Davies C ed (1980) *Rewriting Nursing History* London: Croom Helm

Dean P G (1982) Go ahead, I'm behind you... way behind you. *Socialisation, Sexism and Stereotyping. Women's Issues in Nursing,* ed J Muff. St Louis: C V Mosby

Deaux K (1976) *The Behaviour of Women and Men.* Monterey: Brooks-Cole

de Beauvoir S (1977) *Old Age.* London: Penguin

Deem R (1978) *Women and Schooling.* London: Routledge & Kegan Paul

Department of Employment (1981) *Department of Employment Gazette,* **89**(4) April. London: HMSO

Department of Health and Social Security (1977) *Health and Personal Social Service Statistics for England and Wales.* London: HMSO

Department of Employment (1979) *New Earnings Survey*. London: HMSO

Deutsch H (1945) *The Psychology of Women*. New York: Grune & Stratton

Dickson A (1982) *A Woman in Your Own Right*. London: Quartet

Dingwall R (1979) The place of men in nursing. *Readings in Nursing*, ed M Colledge & M Jones. Edinburgh: Churchill Livingstone

Dunnell K (1979) *Family Formation*. London: Office of Population Censuses and Surveys, HMSO

Dunnell K & Dobbs J (1982) *Nurses Working in the Community*. London: Office of Population Censuses and Surveys, HMSO

Ehrenreich B & English D (1979) *For her Own Good. 100 Years of the Experts' Advice to Women*. London: Pluto Press

Equal Opportunities Commission (1980) *The Experience of Caring for Elderly and Handicapped Dependents*. Manchester: Equal Opportunities Commission

Equal Opportunities Commission (1982a) *Caring for the Elderly and Handicapped: Community Care Policies and Women's Lives*. Manchester: Equal Opportunities Commission

Equal Opportunities Commission (1982b) *Who Cares for the Carers? Opportunities for Those Caring for the Elderly and Handicapped*. Manchester: Equal Opportunities Commission

Fagot B C (1977) Consequences of moderate cross-gender behaviour in pre-school children. *Child Development*, **48**, 902–907

Faust B (1980) *Women, Sexuality and Pornography*. Harmondsworth: Penguin

Finch J & Groves D (1983) *A Labour of Love. Women, Work and Caring*. London: Routledge & Kegan Paul

Foucault M (1977) *Discipline and Punish. The Birth of the Prison*. London: Allen Lane

Fransella F & Frost K (1977) *On Being a Woman*. London: Tavistock Publications

Friedan B (1963) *The Feminine Mystique*. London: Gollancz

Garmarnikov E (1978) Sexual divison of labour: the case of nursing *Feminism and Materialism*, ed A Kuhn and A M Wolpe. London: Routledge & Kegan Paul

Garvey C (1977) *Play*. London: Open Books/Fontana

Gillie O (1981) Sex and cocaine: Freud's pact with the devil. *Sunday Times Weekly Review*, 27 December

Gillie O (1982) The secret love life of Sigmund Freud. *Sunday Times Weekly Review*, 3 January

Glass L & Brand K (1979) The progress of women and nursing: parallel or divergent? *Women in Stress: A Nursing Perspective*, ed D K Kjervik & I M Martinson. New York: Appleton-Century-Crofts

Glucksmann A (1974) Sexual dimorphism in mammals *Biological Review*, **49**, 423–275

Godow A G (1982) *Human Sexuality*. St Louis: C V Mosby

Goffman E (1968) *Asylums*. Harmondsworth: Penguin

Goldsborough J D (1970) On becoming nonjudgemental. *American Journal of Nursing*, November, 2340–2343

Goldthorpe J H, Lockwood D, Bechhofer F & Pratt J (1968) *The Affluent*

Worker: Industrial Attitudes and Behaviour. Cambridge: Cambridge University Press

Gore S (1978) The effect of social support in moderating the health consequences of unemployment. *Journal of Health and Social Behaviour,* **19**(2), 157–165

Gornick V & Moran B eds (1971) *Woman in Sexist Society.* New York: Basic Books

Gove W R & Tudor J F (1972) Adult sex roles and mental illness. *American Journal of Sociology,* **78**, 812–835

Graham H (1984) Caring: a labour of love. *A Labour of Love. Women, Work and Caring,* ed J Finch & D Groves. London: Routledge & Kegan Paul

Gray J A & Drewett R F (1977) The genetics and development of sex differences. *Handbook of Modern Personality Theory,* ed R B Cattell & R M Dreger. New York: Halsted Press

Green R ed (1975) *Human Sexuality: A Health Practitioners' Text.* Baltimore: Williams & Williams

Green J G & Cooke D J (1980) Life stress and symptoms at the climacterium. *British Journal of Psychiatry,* **136**, 486–491

Hartnett D, Boden G & Fuller M eds (1979) *Sex-role Stereotyping.* London: Tavistock Publications

Haug M R & Lavin B (1981) Practitioner or patient – who is in charge? *Journal of Health and Social Behaviour,* **22**(2), 212–229

Heiman, J, LoPiccola L & LoPiccola J (1976) *Becoming Orgasmic. A Sexual Growth Program for Women.* Englewood Cliffs, New Jersey: Prentice-Hall

Hendricks J & Hendricks C D (1978) Sexuality in later life. *An Ageing Population,* ed V Carver & P Liddiard. Sevenoaks: Hodder & Stoughton/ Open University

Henley N & Freeman J (1982) The sexual politics of interpersonal behaviour. *Socialisation, Sexism and Stereotyping. Women's Issues in Nursing,* ed J Muff. St Louis: C V Mosby

Hesselbart S (1977) Women doctors win and male nurses lose. *Sociology of Work and Occupations,* **14**(1), 49–62

Hite S (1976) *The Hite Report.* New York: Macmillan

HMSO (1966) *Report of the Committee on Senior Nursing Staff Structure.* London: HMSO

Hobson D (1978) Housewives: isolation as oppression. *Women Take Issue,* ed Women's Studies Group, Centre for Contemporary Cultural Studies, Birmingham University. London: Hutchinson

Hogan R (1980) *Human Sexuality. A Nursing Perspective.* New York: Appleton-Century-Crofts

Holderby R A & McNulty E G (1982) *Treating and Caring. A Human Approach to Patient Care.* Virginia: Reston

Hotchner B (1980) Menopause and sexuality: gearing up or down? *Topics in Clinical Nursing,* **1**(4), 45–52

Hutt C (1972) *Males and Females.* Harmondsworth: Penguin

Hutter B & Williams G eds (1981) *Controlling Women. The Normal and the Deviant.* London: Croom Helm

Kaplan H S (1978) *The New Sex Therapy.* Harmondsworth: Penguin

Kessler S & McKenna W (1982) Developmental aspects of gender. *The Changing Experience of Women,* ed E Whitelegg *et al.* Oxford: Martin Robertson/Open University

Kinsey A C, Pomeroy W B, Martin C E & Gebhard P H (1948 & 1953) *Sexual Behaviour in the Human Female.* Philadelphia: W B Saunders

Kitzinger S (1962) *The Experience of Childbirth.* London: Gollancz

Kjervik D K & Martinson I M eds (1979) *Women in Stress: A Nursing Perspective.* New York: Appleton-Century-Crofts

Kratz C R ed (1979) *The Nursing Process.* London: Baillière Tindall

Kuczynski H J (1980) Nursing and medical students' sexual attitudes and knowledge. *JOGN Nursing,* Nov–Dec, 339–342

Laws S (1983) The sexual politics of pre-menstrual tension. *Women's Studies International Forum,* **6**(1) 19–31

Lazarus R (1966) *Psychological Stress and the Coping Process.* New York: McGraw-Hill

Lennane K J & Lennane R J (1982) Alleged psychogenic disorders in women. A possible manifestations of sexual prejudice. *The Changing Experience of Women,* ed E Whitelegg *et al.* Oxford: Martin Robertson/Open University

Lief H I (1970) New developments in the sex education of the physician. *Journal of the American Medical Association,* **212** (11), 1864–1867

Lief H I & Payne T (1975) Sexuality – knowledge and attitudes. *American Journal of Nursing,* **75**(11), 2026–2029

Lion E M ed (1982) *Human Sexuality in Nursing Process.* New York: J Wiley

Llewellyn-Jones D (1982) *Everyman.* Oxford: Oxford University Press

Maccoby E E & Jacklin C N (1974) The Psychology of Sex Differences. Stanford: Stanford University Press

Mace D R, Bannerman R H D & Burton J (1974) *The Teaching of Human Sexuality in Schools for Health Professionals.* Geneva: World Health Organisation

MacIntyre S (1976) 'Who wants babies?' The social construction of 'instincts'. *Sexual Divisions in Society: Process and Change* ed D Barker & S Allen. London: Tavistock

MacLeod J ed (1981) *Davidson's Principles and Practice of Medicine.* Edinburgh: Churchill Livingstone

Macleod S (1981) *The Art of Starvation.* London: Virago

Masson J (1984) *Freud: The Assault on Truth.* London: Faber

Masters W H & Johnson V E (1966) *Human Sexual Response.* Boston: Little, Brown & Co

Masters W H & Johnson V E (1970) *Human Sexual Inadquacy.* Boston: Little, Brown & Co

Masters W H & Johnson V E (1979) *Homosexuality in Perspective.* Boston: Little, Brown & Co

McGee M G (1979) Human spatial abilities: psychometric studies and environmental, genetic, hormonal and neurological influences. *Psychological Bulletin,* **86**, 889–918

Menzies I E P (1961) *The Functioning of the Social System as a Defence*

Against Anxiety. London: Tavistock Institute of Human Relations
Meulenbelt A (1981) *For Ourselves: Our Bodies and Sexuality from a Woman's Point of View*. London: Sheba Feminist Publishers
Millman M & Kanter R M (1975) *Another Voice*. New York: Anchor Books
Mitchell J (1979) *Psychoanalysis and Feminism*. New York: Pantheon
Money J & Ehrhardt A A (1972) *Man and Woman, Boy and Girl*. Baltimore: Johns Hopkins University Press
Morris D (1967) *The Naked Ape*. London: Jonathan Cape
Moss H A (1972) Sex, age and state as determinants of mother-infant interaction. *Readings in Child Socialisation*, ed K Danziger. New York: Pergamon
Moyes B (1976) *Perceptions of Pregnancy*. Unpublished PhD thesis: University of Edinburgh
Muff J (1982) Handmaiden, battle-ax, whore: an exploration into fantasies, myths and stereotypes about nurses. *Socialisation, Sexism and Stereotypes. Women's Issues in Nursing*, ed Muff J. St Louis: C V Mosby
Muff J ed (1982) *Socialisation, Sexism and Stereotyping. Women's Issues in Nursing*. St Louis: C V Mosby
Nathanson C A (1975) Illness and the feminine role: a theoretical review. *Social Science & Medicine*, **9**, 57–62
Newson J, Newson E, Richardson D & Scaife J (1978) Perspectives in sex-role stereotyping. *The Sex-role System: Psychological and Sociological Perspectives*, ed J Chetwynd & O Hartnett. London: Routledge & Kegan Paul
Nightingale F (1979) *Cassandra*. New York: Feminist Press
Norbeck J S (1981) Social support; a model for clinical research and application. *Advances in Nursing Science*, July, 43–59
Oakley A (1972) *Sex, Gender and Society*. London: Temple Smith
Oakley A (1974) *The Sociology of Housework*. Oxford: Martin Robertson
Oakley A (1976) Wisewoman and medicine man: changes in the management of childbirth. *The Rights and Wrongs of Women*, ed A Oakley & J Mitchell. Harmondsworth: Penguin
Oakley A (1979) *From Here to Maternity. Becoming a Mother*. Harmondsworth: Penguin
Oakley A (1981) *Subject Women*. Glasgow: Fontana
Oakley A & Mitchell J eds (1976) *The Rights and Wrongs of Women*. Harmondsworth: Penguin
Oakley A, McPherson A & Roberts H (1984) *Miscarriage*. Glasgow: Fontana
Office of Health Economics (1978) *Accidental Deaths. Briefing Pamphlet No 8*. London: Office of Health Economics
Office of Health Economics (1979) *Perinatal Mortality in Britain: A Question of Class. Briefing Pamphlet No 10*. London: Office of Health Economics
Oliver J (1984) The caring wife. *A Labour of Love: Women, Work and Caring*, ed J Finch & D Groves. London: Routledge & Kegan Paul
Oliver J (1983) Letter *The Guardian*, 23 August
Oliver M F (1974) Ischaemic heart disease in young women. *British Medical Journal*, 2 Nov, 253–259

Opit L J (1978) Domiciliarly care for the elderly sick: economy or neglect? *An Ageing Population*, ed V Carver & P Liddiard. Sevenoaks: Hodder & Stoughton/Open University

Orem D (1980) *Nursing: Concepts of Practice*. New York: McGraw-Hill

Parke R D (1979) Perspectives on father-infant interaction. *Handbook of Infancy*, ed J D Osofsky. New York: J Wiley

Payne T (1976) Sexuality of nurses: correlations of knowledge, attitudes and behavior. *Nursing Research*, **25**(4), 286–292

Phillips A & Rakusen J (1979) *Our Bodies, Ourselves*. Harmondsworth: Penguin

Pohl M L (1972) *The Teaching Function of the Nurse Practitioner*. Dubuque, Iowa: W C Brown

Pollock L & West E (1984) On being a woman and a psychiatric nurse. *Senior Nurse*, **1**(17), 10–13

Rambo B J (1984) *Adaptation Nursing. Assessment and Intervention*. Philadelphia: W B Saunders

Redfern S J ed (in press) *Nursing Elderly People*. Edinburgh: Churchill Livingstone

Redman B K (1980) *The Process of Patient Teaching in Nursing*. St Louis: C V Mosby

Reitz R (1981) *Menopause: A Positive Approach*. London: Allen & Unwin

Rheingold H & Cooke K (1975) The contents of boys' and girls' rooms as an index of parents' behavior. *Child Development*, **34**, 1650–1655

Ridgeway V & Mathews A (1982) Psychological preparation for surgery: a comparison of methods. *British Journal of Clinical Psychology*, **21**, 271–289

Riehl J P & Roy C (1980) *Conceptual Models for Nursing Practice*. New York: Appleton-Century-Crofts

Rimmer L (1984) The economics of work and caring. *A Labour of Love. Women, Work and Caring*, ed J Finch & D Groves. London: Routledge & Kegan Paul

Roper N, Logan W W & Tierney A J (1983) *Using a Model for Nursing*. Edinburgh: Churchill Livingstone

Rosenkrantz P S, Vogel S R, Bee H, Broverman I K & Brown D M (1968) Sex-role stereotypes and self-concepts in college students. *Journal of Consulting & Clinical Psychology*, **32**, 287–295

Rosenthal R & Jackson L F (1968) *Pygmalion in the Classroom*. New York: Holt, Rinehart & Winston

Rosser J no date *Becoming a Mother: A Cultural Analysis*. Unpublished research paper, University of Swansea

Royal College of Nursing (1978) *Counselling in Nursing*. The Report of a Working Party held under the Auspices of the RCN Institute of Advanced Nursing Education. London: RCN

Rush F (1984) The great Freudian cover up. *Trouble and Strife*, **4**, 28–36

Russell D (1982) Rape and the masculine mystique. *The Changing Experience of Women*, ed E Whitelegg *et al*. Oxford: Martin Robertson/Open University

Sayers J (1979) On the description of psychological sex differences. *Sex-role Stereotyping,* ed O Hartnett, G Boden & M Fuller. London: Tavistock

Segal L ed (1983) *What is to be Done About the Family?* Harmondsworth: Penguin

Simpson J E P & Levitt R eds (1981) *Going Home.* Edinburgh: Churchill Livingstone

Sisley E L & Harris B (1977) *The Joy of Lesbian Sex.* New York: Mitchell Beazley

Smart C & Smart B eds (1978) *Women, Sexuality and Social Control.* London: Routledge & Kegan Paul

Smythe E E M (1982) Who's going to take care of the nurse? *Socialisation, Sexism and Stereotyping. Women's Issues in Nursing,* ed J Muff. St Louis: C V Mosby

Spender D (1980) *Man-made Language.* London: Routledge & Kegan Paul

Standing H (1980) 'Sickness is a woman's business?': reflections in the attribution of illness. *Alice Through the Looking Glass,* ed L Birke *et al.* London: Virago

Stark E, Flitcraft A & Frazier W (1979) Medicine and patriarchal violence: the social construction of a 'private' event. *International Journal of Health Services,* **9**(3), 461–493

Stein L (1976) The doctor-nurse game. *Archives of General Psychiatry,* **16**, 699–703

Steinmetz SK (1977) Wifebeating, husbandbeating: a comparison of the use of physical violence between spouses to resolve marital fights. *Battered Women: A Psychological Study of Domestic Violence,* ed M Roy. New York: Van Nostrand

Stone G C, Cohen F & Adler N eds (1979) *Health Psychology.* San Francisco: Jossey-Bass

Stuart G W & Sundeen S J eds (1979) *Principles and Practice of Psychiatric Nursing.* St Louis: C V Mosby

Tanner J M (1970) Physical growth. *Carmichael's Manual of Child Psychology. Volume 1* ed P H Mussen. New York: J Wiley

Thomas S (1984) The ten million volunteers question. *The Guardian,* 4 February

Tilly L A & Scott J W (1978) *Women, Work and Family.* New York: Holt, Rinehart & Wilson

Townsend P (1981) Elderly people with disabilities. *Disability in Britain,* ed A Walker & P Townsend. Oxford: Martin Robertson

Tresemer D (1975) Assumptions made about gender roles. *Another Voice,* ed M Millman & R M Kanter. New York: Anchor Books

Tresemer D W (1977) *Fear of Success.* New York: Plenum Press

United Kingdom Central Council for Nursing, Midwifery and Health Visiting (UKCC), PC & R Division (1983) *Code of Professional Conduct for Nurses, Midwives and Health Visitors.* London: UKCC

Versluysen M C (1980) Old wives' tales? Women healers in English history. *Rewriting Nursing History,* ed C Davies. London: Croom Helm

Walker A & Townsend P (1981) *Disability in Britain.* Oxford: Martin Robertson

Webb C (1981) *Changes in Modes of Organisation of Nursing Care.* Unpublished MSc thesis, University of London

Webb C (1982a) Body image and recovery from hysterectomy. *Recovery from Illness,* ed J Wilson-Barnett & M Fordham. Chichester: J Wiley

Webb C (1982b) The men wear the trousers *Nursing Mirror,* **154**(2), 29–31

Webb C (1983) Hysterectomy: dispelling the myths. Parts 1 & 2. *Nursing Times,* Occasional Papers, **79**(30), 52–54 & **79**(31), 44–46

Webb C (1984a) Feminist methodology in nursing research. *Journal of Advanced Nursing,* **9**, 249–256

Webb C (1985a) Nurses' attitudes to therapeutic abortion. *Nursing Times* Occasional Papers, **81**(1), 44–47

Webb C (1985b) Barriers to sympathy. *Nursing Mirror* (Supplement) **160**(1), vi–viii

Webb C (1985c) Gynaecological nursing: a compromising situation. *Journal of Advanced Nursing,* **18**, 47–54.

Webb C (in press) Expressing sexuality. *Nursing Elderly People,* ed S J Redfern. Edinburgh: Churchill Livingstone

Weeks J (1981) *Sexuality, Politics and Society: The Regulation of Sexuality since 1800.* London: Longman

Weg R ed (1983) *Sexuality in Later Years. Roles and Behavior.* New York: Academic Press

Weinberg J S (1982) *Sexuality. Human Needs and Nursing Practice.* Philadelphia: W B Saunders

Weitzman L J, Eifler D, Hokada E & Ross C (Children's Rights Workshop) (1976) *Sex-role Socialisation in Picture Books for Pre-school Children.* London: Writers' and Readers' Publishing Cooperative

Whitelegg E *et al* eds (1982) *The Changing Experience of Women.* Oxford: Martin Robertson/Open University

Williams J H (1977) *Psychology of Women.* New York: Norton & Co

Wilson-Barnett J (1979) *Stress in Hospital.* Edinburgh: Churchill Livingstone

Wilson-Barnett J & Fordham M (1982) *Recovery from Illness.* Chichester: J Wiley

Women's Studies Group, Centre for Contemporary Cultural Studies, Birmingham University (1978) *Women take Issue.* London: Hutchinson

Woods N F ed (1984) *Human Sexuality in Health and Illness.* St Louis: C V Mosby

Worsley P et al (1970) *Introducing Sociology.* Harmondsworth: Penguin

Index